Questions and Answers

in

GENERAL SURGERY

Questions and Answers in GENERAL SURGERY

for revision and self-assessment

H. P. Henderson
FRCS

Senior Registrar, Plastic Surgery,
The Royal Hospital, Sheffield

M. J. Kelly
MChir FRCS MRCP

Senior Surgical Registrar, Royal Devon and
Exeter Hospital, Exeter

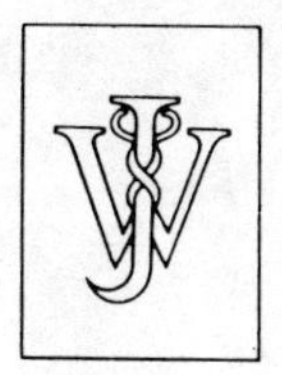

John Wright & Sons Ltd · Bristol 1979

First edition 1979
Reprinted 1980

CIP Data

Henderson, Hugh
Questions & answers in general surgery.
1. Surgery – Problems, exercises etc.
I. Title II. Kelly, Michael J
617'.0076 RD37

ISBN 0 7236 0523 8

Printed in Great Britain by
Billing & Sons Limited, Guildford, London and Worcester

PREFACE

This book arose out of a system of cards that one of us (H.P.H.) used when revising for the final F.R.C.S. examination. Snippets of information were written down in question and answer form on separate cards and carried round in his white coat pocket. This made it possible to indulge in useful revision during any slack moments at work. The collection of questions and answers has been expanded and edited into this small volume which still fits into a white coat pocket.

This book is intended as an aid to relatively painless revision; it is not a comprehensive textbook of surgery. Nothing can take the place of a sound grasp of the contents of the major textbooks reinforced by adequately supervised experience; however revision can also be a problem. The text contains several hundred questions and answers set down in random order; thus an orthopaedic question may follow a neurosurgical one. It is our belief that an ability to provide safe, reasonable, succinct replies on these kind of topics will aid a candidate in the examination and stand him in good stead thereafter.

We believe that candidates should practice answering these questions aloud if possible. This gives good practice at thinking quickly before and while speaking particularly when under the pressure of the examination room. We hope the readers will enlist the help of friends and colleagues to fire these questions at them.

Our aim has been to provide short answers that could be accepted as conforming to the mainstream of current medical practice, and this book stands or falls by the extent to which we have succeeded in this. To this end, we have tried to reference most of our more contentious statements and, for the special departments, we have enlisted the help of the following expert colleagues and friends at the senior registrar and young consultant level.

Arterial Surgery: R. N. Baird, Ch.M., F.R.C.S. Senior Lecturer, Bristol Royal Infirmary.
Bacteriology: R. E. Warren, M.R.C.Path. Consultant Bacteriologist, Addenbrooke's Hospital, Cambridge.

Cardiothoracic Surgery: C. J. Hilton, F.R.C.S. Cardiothoracic Senior Registrar, St. Bartholomew's Hospital, London.
Endocrinology: M. H. Thompson, F.R.C.S. Lecturer, Bristol Royal Infirmary.
E.N.T. Surgery: D. A. Moffat, F.R.C.S. Senior Registrar E.N.T. Dept. The London Hospital.
Gynaecology: C. D. Sims, F.R.C.S., M.R.C.O.G. Queen Charlotte's Hospital, London.
Haematology: C. L. Rist, M.R.C.P. (U.K.) M.R.C.Path. Senior Registrar in Haematology, Bristol Royal Infirmary.
Neurosurgery: C. N. Pidgeon, F.R.C.S.I. Senior Registrar in Neurosurgery, Frenchay Hospital, Bristol.
Orthopaedics: R. G. Grey, F.R.C.S. Senior Registrar, Rowley Bristow Hospital, Pyrford.
Paediatric Surgery: J. D. Frank, F.R.C.S. Senior Registrar, The Hospital for Sick Children, Great Ormond Street, London. and A. E. MacKinnon, F.R.C.S. Consultant Paediatric Surgeon, The Children's Hospital, Sheffield.
Rectal Surgery: M. M. Henry, F.R.C.S. Research Fellow, St. Mark's Hospital, London.
Urology: R. J. Morgan, F.R.C.S. Senior Lecturer, Institute of Urology, St. Peter's Hospitals, London.

H. P. Henderson

M. J. Kelly

FOREWORD

The Right Hon. The Lord Smith of Marlow,K.B.E.,M.S.,F.R.C.S.

The Final F.R.C.S. examination is a good examination in that the examiners expect their successful candidates to display a wide knowledge of surgery in general rather than a high degree of specialised knowledge of the rarities in surgery. Over-all soundness rather than localised brilliance is what is looked for - rightly so when one remembers that essentially this is a test to make certain that those who pass it are ready to be let loose upon an unsuspecting public as surgeons capable, when necessary, of taking decisions on their own responsibility and of acting upon them.

Candidates who possess this corpus of general surgical knowledge and experience will nearly always pass the examination, but not necessarily at the first attempt, for every examination has its own particular flavour and demands its own style and technique if success is to follow, and the Final Fellowship is no exception. That is why it is not unusual for a candidate whose knowledge is perfectly adequate nevertheless to present his wares less well than he might and to need perhaps one "trial run" before he gets the hang of the examination and passes it at the second attempt.

How nice it would be if one could have this trial run "for free", as it were - if one could get it over in advance before sitting the examination for the first time.

Well, of course, one can't; but one could, I suppose, get near it if, as a potential candidate, one were allowed unlimited access as an observer, a "fly on the wall", at the viva voce examinations of all the candidates at many Final F.R.C.S. examinations. Here again, the chances of the Court of Examiners acquiescing in such a scheme are remote, so the whole idea is a pipe-dream - or is it?

The Authors of this book have sought, in a concise and readable form, to provide for its reader questions and answers conveying unmistakably the flavour of the Final Fellowship and they have succeeded admirably in doing so. As an introduction to what candidates may expect in the examination, the style of questioning and the depths of knowledge expected, it is immensely informative and as a source of surgical revision, to dip into when opportunities for sustained reading are few, it succeeds where more formal textbooks necessarily fail.

Is it then just a "crammer's" book, useful only in order to pass one particular examination? It would be unjust to criticise it on this score. As I have written above, the Final F.R.C.S.is a good examination and a study of the questions asked in it cannot be pursued without absorbing a wealth of surgical knowledge essential to a successful career in surgery. That is why this book should surely be a possession not only of candidates about to sit the Final F.R.C.S. for the first time but also their more senior colleagues as well - including the examiners!

March, 1979 SMITH.

Practice Essay Questions

We believe that it is worthwhile writing out at least two or three essays in full before the written paper, to practice timing and organising your thoughts on paper. If this discipline seems too great then at least practice writing out the important headings or key words that must be included. In regard to the essay paper the advice of one of us (H.P.H.) is to first write out the outline headings of all the questions on scrap paper; then to answer the question which seems easiest and most straightforward, during which time the brain can be unconsciously thinking about the question or questions that don't seem so easy, and additions can be made to the outline headings of the latter.

a) Discuss the pathology and treatment of osteoarthritis.

b) Give a brief description of the embryology of the ureter, and describe the management of malignant ureteric neoplasms.

c) Discuss the control of infection in operating theatre suites.

d) How would you manage a 60 year old patient in whom you detect a carcinoma of rectum on out-patient sigmoidoscopic examination?

e) List the uses, abuses, and resultant complications of corticosteroid administration in surgical patients.

f) Describe the different modes of presentation, methods of diagnosis, and treatment of aneurysms of the aorta just above the bifurcation.

g) What is the management of a young motor cyclist brought to Casualty with a suspected fractured skull?

h) Discuss the treatment of electrical burns.

i) Compare the pathology of ulcerative colitis and Crohn's disease of the large bowel.

j) Describe the anatomy of the femoral canal, and describe one surgical technique of treating a strangulated femoral hernia.

k) Discuss the rationale of the different methods available for preventing Deep Vein Thrombosis.

l) Write an essay on the management of lymphoedema of the leg.

1 What are the commoner causes of acquired fistula between intestine and vagina?

2 In assessing a patient with claudication for possible surgery what other medical points in a general history are noteworthy?

3 A 10 years old coloured boy presents with severe central abdominal pain. Are there any special preoperative blood tests that you ought to do?

4 Who introduced the abdomino-perineal resection of the rectum and why?

5 Cytomegalic inclusion disease)
Hypoparathyroidism) have what in common?
Sturge-Weber Syndrome)

6 On clinical examination, which benign conditions may simulate a testicular tumour?

7 What is the treatment of a poorly differentiated carcinoma of the nasopharynx with metastatic nodes palpable?

8 What is unusual about the bleeding associated with diverticular disease?

1 a) Inflammatory disease eg Crohn's, UC, diverticular d., *L. venereum*

b) Malignant disease

c) Irradiation

d) Operative trauma and infection

2 History of angina, cerebrovascular accident, diabetes or hypertension. Details of smoking habits and past history with reference to fitness for a long general anaesthetic.

3 Yes: a) Sickle cell test

b) Hb, (it will be low in thalassaemia)

c) (G6PD deficiency test might be desirable, but it takes many hours to do)

4 Sir Ernest Miles in about 1907. He had reviewed cases of rectal cancer and was appalled by the high recurrence rate following the then current practice of local excision. He postulated downward, lateral and upward spread of rectal cancer which necessitated en bloc excision of the anus and rectum.

5 Intra-cranial calcification

6 Haematocele, granulomatous orchitis, sperm granuloma, any chronic orchitis, cyst of the testis.
If in <u>any</u> doubt, explore through an inguinal approach using a soft clamp on the cord as you deliver the testicle.

7 External irradiation using supervoltage and including the cervical nodes followed sometimes by neck dissection for residual operable disease. (Although the latter adds little to the survival figures).

8 It is commoner in diverticulosis than diverticulitis. It may cause a major loss of blood requiring transfusion.

9 What does $T_{4b}N_3M_1$ tumour of the breast mean?

10 What size tube should you be sure is available before you start to do a tracheostomy?

11 You are asked to write an essay on the management of the diabetic foot. Write down the headings you would use to cover this subject.

9 T_4 = A tumour of any size which extends directly to the chest wall or skin.

T_{4b} = As above, with oedema, infiltration, of the skin including peau d'orange or satellite skin nodules confined to the same breast.

N_3 = Ipsilateral supraclavicular or infraclavicular nodes involved or oedema of the arm.

M_1 = Distant metastases present, including skin involvement beyond the breast area.

It is equivalent to "Stage IV"

10 In men probably a Portex size 36-40 or Silver size 34-36.
In women probably a Portex size 30-36 or Silver 30-32.
In children have a wide range available.

11 History and examination with particular reference to....
Investigations (including Full blood count, electrolytes, sugar levels. X-rays. Chest and Arteriography if appropriate. Ankle pressure measurement, fibrinogen level (viscosity).

Treatment (Divide this up into general and local, medical and surgical)

General: Diabetic control, nutrition, treatment of heart, chest and eyes. Vitamin replacement, control of alcoholism, and smoking if appropriate.

Local: Control of sepsis. Mechanical debridement, local amputation of digit or ray, eradication of ostemyelitis. Use of systemic or local antiobiotics/ antiseptics. Skin grafting of ulcers.

Improvement in circulation:

Medical: Physiotherapy; Lumbar sympathectomy (discuss value of it)
Fibrinogen reducing drugs - clofibrate; Vasodilators.

Surgical: Reconstructive procedures

Protection of the foot: Special dressings, appliances, footwear chiropody.

Complications: failure of local treatment - discuss levels of amputation.

Follow-up.

12 In a case of suspected arterial embolism to a limb what are the danger signs of irreversible ischaemia?

13 In what clinical situations is hyperbaric oxygen of use?

14 What are the layers of the wall of a hydatid cyst?

15 About 25% of patients with carcinoid tumours have something else wrong with them - what?

16 What may the patient with chondromalacia patellae complain of?

17 If you choose to treat all spina bifida cases however serious their disability, what % can you expect to end up earning a living and leading reasonably independent lives?

12 a) Sensory Loss (By far the best prognostic guide)
b) Waxy pallor
c) Temperature loss
d) Muscle weakness, tenderness or rigidity

13 Carbon monoxide poisoning
Air embolism
Decompression sickness
Gas gangrene
Operative management of some cases of cyanotic heart disease
Some cases of severe hypoxaemia due to pulmonary disease
Occasionally post-operatively for pulmonary complications

14 Outer: pseudocyst (fibrous coat of host reaction)
Middle: ectocyst
Inner: endocyst (germinal lining layer)

An uninfected hydatid cyst has a pellucid membranous covering and contains clear fluid

15 Another malignant neoplasm

16 Pain on ascending stairs; discomfort on prolonged sitting with knees flexed; inability to kneel without pain: occasionally swelling of the knee joint; the knee may 'give way'.
(N.B. The knee will not lock unless there is a loose body within it)

17 About 10% (See Lorber's papers. *British Medical Journal 1973. iv. 201*

18 What non-neoplastic benign tumours (inflammatory, traumatic and degenerative) occur in the larynx?

19 What is 'Saint's Triad'?

20 Increased intracranial pressure due to simple head injury may be early or late. Distinguish between the two.

21 Apart from the gut in what other organs may carcinoids be found?

22 What infection may be found in a Chinaman who presents with pain pyrexia, jaundice, bile in the urine and, occasionally, clay-coloured stools?

23 What % of patients with Crohn's disease respond usefully to azathiaprine?

24 What is the commonest site of osteochondritis dissecans?

25 How would you treat a small primary of anterior 1/3 of the tongue with a unilateral node?

18 Singer's nodes (usually bilateral, occur at junction of ant. 1/3 and post 2/3 of vocal cords)

Chronic laryngitis (Reinkes subepithelial oedema)

Intubation granuloma

Tuberculous laryngitis

Syphilitic laryngitis

Wegener's granuloma

Retention cysts

Amyloidosis

19 Gall-stones
Diverticulitis
Hiatus Hernia

20 Immediate increased pressure is related to expansion of the vascular bed secondary to vasoparesis, itself often due to hypoxia. Hence the importance of the airway in head injuries. Later increased press re, if haematoma formation is excluded, may be due to true brain oedema. The advent of direct pressure monitoring has improved management of this.

21 Bronchus, pancreas, gall-bladder, ovary, testis.

22 Commonly *Clornorchis sinensis* (*liver fluke*).
Specialist advice and treatment indicated.

23 33% respond dramatically for as long as it is continued, but most relapse when it is stopped *(Leonard Jones and Williams, Proceedings of the Royal Society of Medicine (1972) 65, 291-3)*

24 The lateral side of the medial femoral condyle.

25 Wide local excision - v-shape - and construction of new tongue tip and unilateral radical neck dissection.

26 A patient requiring prostatectomy says that he has a bleeding tendency. Which laboratory tests would you order?

27 What kinds of head injuries predispose to late epilepsy?

28 What are the three basic stages described by McKeown in the operation of oesophagectomy for Ca Oesophagus? (See B.J.S. (1976) 63.259-262.)

29 What is the use of methylprednisolone in transplant patients?

30 What are the radiographic signs seen on peripheral arteriograms which suggest malignancy of bone or soft tissue tumours?

31 Describe the anatomy of Stensen's Duct

32 Often in transplanted kidneys only the tips of minor calyces are visible on I.V.U. Why is this?

33 What are the normal intra-cardiac pressures? (Each chamber)

26 Prothrombin Time, APPT, Thrombin Clotting Time, Bleeding Time
Platelet count

27 Those with:

1) A post-traumatic amnesia of more than 24 hours
2) Early post-traumatic epilepsy
3) A depressed fracture with dural tearing or focal signs

28
1) Abdominal stage to mobilise the stomach
2) A Right thoracotomy to excise the oesophagus
3) A Right cervical incision to perform the oesophago-gastric anastomosis

29 It may be useful in treatment of acute rejection and late onset rejection

30
a) Pathological vessels not conforming to normal anatomy
b) Abrupt termination of large vessels near the tumour or at its periphery due to thrombosis
c) Abnormal venous lakes and large draining veins, with early venous filling

31 It emerges from the anterior border of the parotid gland close to the branch of the VIIth nerve to the alae nasi and is crossed itself by the transverse facial artery. It then lies on the masseter and pierces the buccinator to emerge beneath the mucous membrane of the mouth opposite the second upper molar.

32 It may be impossible for the radiographer to apply pressure over the ureters

33 Right Atrium: $\frac{+2}{-2}$ Left Atrium: $\frac{+3}{0}$

Right Ventricle: $\frac{30}{1}$ Left Ventricle: $\frac{120}{0}$

Pulmonary Artery: $\frac{30}{15}$

34 Radiological widening of the skull sutures and a 'copper-beaten' appearance indicate what?

35 Metastatic spread is likely to be clinically detected in which groups of lymph nodes from a carcinoma of the posterior 1/3 of the tongue?

36 What is the common post-operative complications in a baby who has had a laparotomy for meconium ileus?

37 Malignant change in Paget's disease of bone generally leads to what kind of tumour?

38 What is the usual final position of the femur in the untreated severely osteoarthritic hip?

39 What is the commonest cause of subclavian vein thrombosis?

40 What is the main difference in the electrolyte balance seen in patients with an ileo-rectal anastomosis and patients with an ileostomy?

41 What is the action of lactulose as an aperient? (50% lactulose 5 ml once or twice daily).

42 Relapse of which tropical disease usually controllable by drugs is made much more frequent and serious after splenectomy?

43 When does a simple goitre become irreversible?

34 Raised intra-cranial pressure in a child. N.B. In the adult raised I.C.P. leads to erosion of the posterior clinoid processes.

35 Jugulo-digastric group of upper deep cervical lymph nodes (often bilateral).

36 Pulmonary infection due to Cystic fibrosis.

37 Usually osteosarcoma, but it can be fibrosarcoma.

38 Adducted, flexed and externally rotated.

39 Unusual exercise of the arm. (The thrombosis is usually located in the region between the clavicle and Ist rib).

40 The ileostomy patient is relatively more dehydrated and shows greater sodium loss in the faeces and hence Sodium deficiency.

41 Lactulose is a synthetic dissacharide and has no direct action on the bowel mucosa or its innervation. When taken orally it reaches the colon mostly unaltered and is broken down by saccharolytic flora with increased production of lactic acid and other organic acids. This is said to encourage normal propulsive movements.

42 Malaria.

43 At the stage of nodularity.

44 Give some causes of single rarified areas in bones on X-Ray examination.

45 Dextrocardia may be one of the apparent clinical findings on examination of a new-born infant in respiratory distress. What surgically correctable condition may be the cause?

What is the immediate management of such a condition?

46 Through which side of the chest would you do a thoracotomy for an oesophageal tear?

47 Continuous anal pain, a lump in the wall of the anal canal, with history of bleeding or discharge, characterises what condition which is not a perianal haematoma nor abscess nor thrombosed pile?

48 Give a classification of goitre.

49 What is the site of election for a forearm amputation?

44 Solitary cysts (disappear after puberty)
Cysts associated with osteoarthritis of a joint
Inflammation (T.B., Brodie's abscess)
Tumour: benign - chondroma, giant cell tumour, granuloma
malignant - sarcoma of lytic type, isolated secondary neoplasm.

45 A diaphragmatic hernia of the Left sided Bochdalek type.

a) Pass naso-gastric tube to deflate the stomach and suck out swallowed air

b) Give O_2

c) Endotracheal intubation and <u>gentle</u> ventilation - (rupture of an alveolus can lead to pneumothorax).

46 If it is near the cardia, perform the thoractomy on the side that the patient has either the pneumothorax, effusion or pain. On the whole it is easier to approach other parts of the oesophagus through a Right Thoracotomy.

47 Intersphinteric abscess. Treatment is to lay it open; (it may be caused by infection of an anal gland as a stage of development of a fistula in ano) See Parks *B.J.S. (1976) 63 1 - 12.*

48 Simple: Endemic, sporadic, diffuse hyperplastic, nodular.
Toxic: Diffuse toxic (Graves), toxic nodular goitre, toxic nodule.
Neoplastic: follicular, papillary anaplastic, medullary, benign.
Thyroiditis: granulomatous, autoimmune (Hashimoto's), Reidel's.
Rarities: Acute bacterial thyroiditis, chronic bacterial thyroiditis (T.B. Syphilis) amyloid.

49 Between 15-18 cm below the tip of the adult olecranon.

50 What do the following have in common:- Fragilitas ossium, Nail-Patella syndrome, Achondroplasia, Diaphyseal Aclasis, Dupuytren's Contracture, Marfan's syndrome?

51 What is the action of Sodium Warfarin or Phenindione?

52 What does aphakic mean?

53 What are the indications for emergency craniotomy?

54 What is a ranula?

55 What are the main indications for endarterectomy rather than by-pass grafting in lower limb ischaemia?

56 How do you control the blood supply to the upper pole in a partial thyroidectomy?

50 A dominant inheritance pattern.

51 These inhibit liver synthesis of the normal plasma proteins which are Vitamin K dependent clotting factors. i.e. Prothrombin and factors VII, IX and X. (Thus Prothrombin time rises).

52 Without lens (Post cataract extraction for example).

53 The principal indication is rapidly rising intracranial pressure due to a mass lesion. Localization may be unreliable without specialist radiology. A head injury deteriorating too rapidly to allow transfer is the only common indication for non-specialist intervention. A haematoma may be sought by burr holes and when found, a craniectomy or craniotomy done to improve evacuation.

54 A cystic swelling in the floor of the mouth. It is usually due to cystic degeneration of a mucous or salivary gland. It is often difficult to remove. Marsupialisation may be the easiest way of dealing with it.

55 Some surgeons always prefer by-pass grafting because long term results of endarterectomy are disappointing, however endarterectomy may be appropriate if the stenosis is relatively short and affects a large artery such as an iliac artery. Other lesser reasons include lack of a suitable saphenous vein for by-pass, or if dacron grafts are inappropriate, or if the patient's condition is poor and a long operation is inadvisable.

56 The classic way is to insinuate a Kocher's grooved director deep to the upper pole in which lie the superior thyroid vessels. Ensure that the director is superficial to the cricothyroid and the external laryngeal nerve. Doubly ligate the upper pole leaving 5 mm cuff of tissue distal to the ligature. Many surgeons use a transfixion suture for one of these ligatures. Loss of control of the upper pole is a serious error which can be technically difficult to retrieve.

57 Which flexor tendon in the hand most commonly ruptures in severe advanced rheumatoid disease?

58 Meconium ileus is the neonatal manifestation of what disease?

59 What is the main contraindication to the axillary approach for cervical sympathectomy?

60 How would you assess clinically a patient brought into casualty with a head injury?

61 What is the commonest cause of incompatible blood transfusion?

62 What is the Boari flap operation?

63 What is the action of Heparin?

64 What is Meigs' syndrome, and how may it present to the general surgeon?

57 F.P.L. (Flexor pollicis longus)

58 Fibrocystic disease.

59 Evidence of adhesions at the lung apex making a transpleural approach difficult.

60 After the initial recussitative sequence, the following are assessed and recorded:

1) The level of conciousness
2) Posture, movements and reflexes
3) Eye movements and pupils
4) Any gross focal deficit.

Any evidence of change in the above is of particular significance. A thorough general examination and search for other injury should also be made.

61 Clerical error.

62 A full thickness triangular flap of bladder wall is raised (based on the dome with apex from the anterior bladder) and this flap is tubed to create a conduit to which a shortened ureter can be anastomosed without any tension.

63 In low doses it combines with Anti-Thrombin III and inhibits activated FactorX. At this concentration it may inhibit thrombosis but has little effect on the whole blood clotting time. In higher doses it combines with not only Anti-Thrombin III but thrombin itself and prevents the conversion of fibrinogen to fibrin.

64 Meigs' syndrome is the presence of a pleural effusion, left or right sided, ascites and an ovarian fibroma. Removal of the affected ovary cures the condition. The patient may present with respiratory problems or lower abdominal pain due to torsion of the ovary.

65 What is the underlying principle in the posterior extrapleural approach to draining a subphrenic abscess?

66 List some of the important factors which influence the outcome of arterial surgery for chronic arterial occlusion?

67 What is Muir's tube?

68 Describe aloud as in the operative part of your viva how you would perform an elective splenectomy.

65 The method depends upon the ability to strip the parietal pleura off the ribs at the costo-diaphragmatic angle, after resection of the tenth rib, thereby getting above the liver and incising the abscess extrapleurally. However local inflamation may make this stripping very difficult.

66 It is always better to operate on Localised disease, in a Large artery, Free of calcification, in a Clean field, in a young, non-diabetic, patient who is in Good general health and free of Heart disease, and not Obese, who is prepared to give up Smoking, and who has a compelling disability with a bad prognosis if left untreated. Reconstruction should use autogenous material in preference to foreign, and be done by an experienced surgeon rather than an inexperienced one.

67 A glass tube with a side piece for irrigation of bowel peroperatively, connecting the bowel to some Paul's tubing.

68 A fully prepared, properly investigated patient is taken to the operating theatre. Two units of blood have been cross-matched. The patient is anaesthetised and place supine on the operating table, with facility for right lateral tilt. The skin is prepared and suitably draped. I would make a left paramedian incision (or subcostal or midline incision). After initial laparotomy I would pass my hand up and over the lateral aspect of the spleen, grasp it gently and draw it across into the wound. I'd divide avascular adhesions by sharp and blunt dissection and then attempt division of its posterior attachment (the lieno-renal ligament) taking great care not to damage the vessels. I should then cut the gastro-splenic ligament between ligatures to secure the short gastric blood vessels being careful not to injure the left colic flexure or stomach. Next I'd expose the main splenic vessels from behind, holding the spleen medially and gently pushing the tail of the pancreas out of the way, I'd pass a finger around the vascular pedicle, clamp, and doubly tie the artery and vein(s) separately. Before closing the abdomen after removing the spleen I'd check for accessory spleens and, if satisfied with haemostasis and that stomach, spleen and colon were undamaged, would close without drainage. If in doubt I would insert a drain to lie in the splenic bed. (Be prepared to justify your chosen incision.)

69 Which bacteria may produce the clinical picture of acute appendicitis, but at laparotomy the appendix appears to be normal?

70 How long a history attributable to diverticular disease is given by 80% of those patients who die directly from it?

71 In general, which types of anaerobic infections fail to respond to hyperbaric oxygen therapy?

72 How do you control the blood supply to the lower pole in a partial thyroidectomy?

73 What is the site of election for amputation of the humerus?

74 A healthy child or adult complains of intermittent attacks of central abdominal pain unrelated to any obvious precipitating cause. These attacks may occur at intervals of weeks or months, sometimes with vomiting, and nearly always terminate with diarrhoea ± blood. The pain is usually acute in onset, severe, lasting for 2-3 days gradually fading. Abdominal distension is usually not a notable feature of the clinical examination during such an attack. What is the likely cause, and what single investigation might give the diagnosis?

75 You are shown a 'Pot' of the heart. In one of the cardiac chambers you see a firm globular mass or soft polypoid mass. What is it likely to be - and which chamber is it most likely to occupy?

69 i) *Salmonella* and *Shigella sonnei* infections can mimic appendicitis (diagnosis by stool culture).

ii) *Yersinea pseudotuberculosis* rarely produces a terminal ileitis with mesenteric adenitis, (diagnosis by culture of mesenteric node, stool and serum agglutination tests).

70 Less than a month.

71 The non-clostridial ones. In fact, an early response to hyperbaric oxygen is said to be indicative of clostridial infection.

72 Ligation and division of the inferior thyroid veins,and ligation in continuity of the inferior thyroid artery well laterally to avoid damage to the recurrent laryngeal nerve.

73 Optimally 18-20 cm below the acromion in the adult.

74 A midgut malrotation. Barium meal and follow through.

75 Myxoma - Left Atrium.

76 Why is early surgery attempted in the treatment of ruptured intra-cranial aneurysms?

77 How did John Hunter describe the stomach?

78 Whose name is associated with superficial thrombophlebitis anywhere along the line from the antecubital fossa through the axilla and obliquely down to the umbilicus? (It may or may not be painful; may be due to trauma or malignant disease and is usually self-limiting resolving spontaneously.)

79 In whom is a retropharyngeal abscess likely to occur?

80 Which lymph node groups are removed in a block dissection of the neck?

81 When does ectopic pregnancy usually rupture?

82 Having explored, confirmed and dealt with a testicular torsion, what should you do next?

83 What sort of substance is L.A.T.S.? How important is it as a cause of disease?

76 Without treatment there is an approximate mortality of 50% within six months. Recurrence of haemorrhage is commonest in the first six weeks post-bleed. Surgical mortality is high in patients in poor neurological condition. Results of emergency surgery are poor. Given good patient condition, surgery between five and ten days post bleeding is optimal. While awaiting surgery, rebleeding may be reduced by antifibrinolytics.

77 The stomach is a gland with a cavity.

78 Mondor's Disease. It may sometimes be mistaken for a breast lump.

79 In children less than five years of age following an upper respiratory tract infection and as a complication of retropharyngeal lymphadenopathy leading to an acute abscess: the chronic type generally follows T.B. of the spine. However, the latter usually tracks laterally posterior to the prevertebral fascia and points behind the posterior margin of S/mastoid.

80 Submental, submandibular, upper and lower deep cervical, anterior and supraclavicular and nodes in post Δ.

81 Rupture commonly occurs at 4-8th week of amenorrhoea. It depends on the site of implantation. Ectopics in the narrow tubal isthmus rupture early, whereas those in the wide ampulla cause problems late.

82 Fix the other side. Some surgeons prefer to delay this by 2-3 weeks, but most fix the other side at the same operation.

83 Probably IgG antibody, but no corresponding antigen has been found for it. L.A.T.S. may be an important factor in the cause of Grave's disease, but the evidence is far from complete.

84 You are shown a very obvious Charcot joint as a short examination case, and you are given a couple of minutes to examine the rest of the patient; what systems and things should you immediately and without hesitation examine?

85 What instructions should you give about the handling of a severed part such as a foot or a finger in the time taken between the first casualty assessment and definitive surgical treatment?

86 Where does the middle rectal artery arise, and what does it supply in the male?

87 Should diabetic patients undergoing upper leg amputations be given antibiotics and, if so, which, when and why?

88 What is the action of aspirin on platelet behaviour?

84 Think first of the causes:

Syphilis: Check eyes for Argyll Robertson pupils, heart for aortic incompetence, perform a Romberg test, look at the abdomen for scars of surgery done in tabetic crisis, and test Achilles tendon deep pain sensation. Also look at skin trophic changes, and test lower limb reflexes (for loss).

Diabetes Mellitus: Peripheral neuropathy and ischemia. Ask the patient if diabetic!

Syringomyelia: Look for dissociated sensory loss.

Peripheral neuropathy:

85 Tell the person responsible for the severed part to place it within a clean unused (but not necessarily sterile) plastic bag, and to seal the plastic bag with tape. Then to place this plastic bag within another containing ice. Emphasize that the part should not be soaked in antiseptic or antibiotic, that canulation of vessels should be resisted, and finally do not plunge the part directly into an ice bucket - water damages exposed tissues.

86 It arises either from the internal iliac or the inferior vesical artery. It runs medially to the rectum giving branches also to the prostate, seminal vesicles, and ductus deferens. It supplies mainly muscle of the ampulla rather than the mucosa and does not anastomose with the superior rectal artery directly.

87 YES ALWAYS

i) The risk of gas gangrene is high. Benzyl penicillin 1 - 2 Megaunits 4 - 6 hourly is the drug of choice against all *Clostridia*. Treatment should start with the premedication and continue for at least five days to allow for revascularisation.

ii) Local pyogenic sepsis is usually due to *Staph. aureus*, and is best covered by flucloxacillin. *Leading article, British Medical Journal 1969 I 665 - 6.*

88 It may contribute to inhibition of aggregation and it does affect platelet adhesiveness.

89 What is a sentinel pile associated with?

90 What % of patients with rectal carcinoma come into the Duke's A category?

91 What is the treatment of a carcinoma of the floor of the mouth or lip with no obvious metastatic disease?

92 What does S.O.S. mean pharmaceutically speaking?

93 How much blood is it advisable to culture in an adult to diagnose Gram-negative septicaemia?

89 Classically the sentinel pile occupies one end of a chronic fissure. It may be sentinel to a rectal carcinoma lying above it.

90 About 15% (Duke's B - about 35% and Duke's C - about 50%) *(Bailey and Love). Lockhart-Mummery, Ritchie and Hawley B.J.S. (1976) 63 673-7.*

91 Either A: excision of primary followed by prophylactic X.R.T. (about 5,000 rads in five weeks) or

B: excision of primary and if metastatic nodes appear give X.R.T. (6,000 rads) then radical N. dissection.

This is controversial, but another reasonable treatment plan is:

i) floor of mouth - surgery and partial mandibulectomy and bone graft reconstruction. (No D.X.T. at all).
anterior floor of mouth - surgery and partial mandibulectomy and bone graft reconstruction and bilateral suprahyoid neck dissection (if histologically involved nodes then proceed to radical neck dissection). No D.X.T.

ii) Lip - excision of primary - if metastatic nodes appear, D.X.T. then radical neck dissection if the nodes do not resolve.

92 Si opus sit (Latin = if the matter should be, i.e. if necessary)

93 A minimum of 20 ml. This increases the positive diagnosis rate by up to 30% compared to a 10 ml culture. *(Hall et al. 1976 J.Clin.Microbiol. 3 643-645).* In half of Gramnegative Septicaemias there have been less than 1 colony- forming unit per ml of blood. *(Finegold in Bacteria pub. CC Press 1974).*

94 Describe a through knee amputation - operative technique.

95 What are the important contraindications to prostatectomy?

96 In the follow-up of a patient after partial gastrectomy, what blood tests whould be done?

97 What % of polyps can be seen radiologically in the colon by using a double contrast enema?

98 Which Parotid tumour tends to spread peri-neurally?

94 The patient is anaesthetised and placed supine on the table with the leg hanging over the end of the table. The incisions are marked out to give a long anterior flap to below the level of the tibial tubercle, and short posterior flap at the level of the joint line. The incision lines meet at an angle overlying the posterior aspects of the lateral femoral condyles. Incise the skin of the anterior flap down to periosteum and elevate the flap. Divide the insertion of ligamentum patellae, quadriceps expansion, and collateral and cruciate ligaments leaving the latter long for ease of later suture. Then either lift the leg or turn the patient over to gain ready access to the posterior aspect. The posterior incision is now made and deepened and the popliteal artery and vein ligated and divided. The popliteal nerve is divided high up. The hamstring muscles are divided at the level of the joint line. As much synovial tissue is removed from the intercondylar notch as possible and the patellar tendon is sutured to the cruciates. The patella should lie in its normal position on the femur, not pulled around. The hamstrings are then attached to the cruciates and capsular tissue and fascia lata repaired. Drains are inserted before skin closure. A firm bandage is applied. Post-operatively the patient is encouraged to use an ischial bearing pylon until the wound is healed. He is then fitted with an end bearing closely fitted socket prosthesis. The advantage of this stump lies in its asymmetry; the prosthesis cannot rotate.

95 a) A mentally deranged patient who is unlikely to co-operate in the post-operative period.

b) The patient is unfit for any form of general or regional anaesthesia.

96 Full blood count: detects anaemia (iron or B12 deficiency)

Serum iron and iron binding capacity

B12 level

Ca and Ca/alb levels.

97 About 95% of polyps over 5mm diameter.

98 Adenoid cystic carcinoma) both spread perineurally
Cylindroma)

99 Give an outline list of the causes of Post-operative Pyrexia.

100 Which organism is frequently the cause of skin graft failure, and which actually destroys the graft? If such an organism is cultured from a patient's wound before or after grafting, what action should be taken?

101 Do you consider that arterial patients should be required to 'earn' their amputation?

102 In the Zollinger-Ellison Syndrome what effect on the plasma gastrin level would you expect with the secretin and calcium infusion tests?

99 Infection: Operation site
Wound
Chest
Urine — Catheter; Instrumentation Bacteraemia

D.V.T.
Drugs < Anaesthetic (Halothane Sensitivity etc.); Antibiotics

Blood Haematoma
Transfusion Reaction

100 Haemolytic *Streptococcus*, Lancefield Group A.
The patient must be isolated if the lesion is extensive. If he is about to undergo operation, it should be postponed. Benzyl penicillin is the drug of choice or, if there is a concomitant *Staph aureus*, give flucloxacillin.
Search for the source of the *Streptococcus* in the patient (nose, throat) and ward staff and consult microbiologist about further measures.

101 The precept of 'earning an amputation' overstates the argument to make the case. Except when patients are too confused by the toxic effects of peripheral gangrene to make a rational decision, it is most unwise to press for an amputation in the absence of severe symptoms. Patients who feel that they have had an amputation forced on them seldom try hard to rehabilitate themselves with a prosthesis, and may bear a grudge against the surgeon, making management of the patient very difficult. Nevertheless, under the right circumstances, amputation is a good operation leading to rapid healing and rehabilitation.

102 Secretin test: large rise in gastrin (normal falls or slight rise)

Calcium infusion: gastrin doubles (normal may rise too, even quite high)

103 What are the main indications for prostatectomy?

104 What information does measuring gentamicin levels give in a seriously ill patient?

105 List some of the indications for total intravenous nutrition in a child.

106 Why was the carcinoid tumour called thus?

107 What are the probable causes of chocolate coloured fluid in the peritoneal cavity?

103 a) one or more attacks of acute urinary retention with inability to void after catheter withdrawal.

b) chronic retention with overflow incontinence.

c) symptoms of poor stream and/or disabling frequency (provided this is not associated with bladder instability).

d) recurrent or persistent urinary tract infection associated with a large residual post-micturitional volume.

e) vesical stone formation associated with bladder neck obstruction.

104 (i) In renal impairment, a level above 2 mg/l immediately before another dose suggests accumulation and the consequent need to repeat the levels to guide dosage and avoid toxicity.

(ii) In all situations, evidence that adequate dosage is being given. Underdosage is common. Levels 1 hour after i.m., and ¼ hour after i.v. dosage should exceed 5 mg/l in non pulmonary infections, and be more than 8 mg/l in pneumonia due to Gram neg. organisms.

105 Extensive bowel resection
Recurrent intestinal obstruction
Intestinal fistulae
Prolonged ileus
Malabsorption states i.e. following prolonged diarrhoea

106 It was thought to be benign despite histology more indicative of malignancy.
Benign carcinoids can occur in the appendix.
Other carcinoids are all potentially malignant, although metastases from rectal carcinoids are rare.
About 1/3 carcinoids have metastases.

107 Thick milk chocolate-type fluid is due to endometriosis.
Thinner fluid may be caused by retrograde menstruation
or ruptured ovarian cyst with blood
or pelvic colon volvulus.

108 How common is co-existent osteoarthritis of the hip in cases of subcapital and transcervical fractured neck of femur?

109 You have operated on a 22 year old unmarried woman for appendicitis and find a ruptured right tubal ectopic pregnancy. What would you do at operation?

110 In what bowel disease are nerve trunks seen between the muscle layers in the absence of ganglion cells?

111 Bolt distinguishes two types of peritonitis in acute diverticular disease. What are these?
Bolt D.E., Diverticular Disease of the Large Intestine 1973 Annals R.C.S.E. <u>*53*</u> *237-245*

112 What surgical procedures should be done in a staging laparotomy for Hodgkin's disease?

108 Very rare indeed. (Probably less than 1% of cases of fractured neck of femur have osteoarthritis): because of the thickening of the neck which osteoarthritis produces. Trochanteric fractures in osteoarthritis are not as rare.

109 Suck out free blood and clots and identify the bleeding Fallopian tube. Place clamps proximally and distally to control haemorrhage. Now inspect the other side, with enlargement of the wound if necessary. If the other tube and ovary appear normal excise the affected tube. If the other tube is damaged, conserve as much of the affected right tube as possible with a view to later reconstructive surgery. If in doubt obtain expert assistance.

110 Hirschsprung's.

111 a) Turbid or purulent peritonitis: the patient has a toxic illness with fever, tachycardia, lower abdominal tenderness, guarding, peritonism and diminished bowel sounds. These patients probably have ruptured a peri-colic abscess and there is no free open perforation. The bowel is inflamed and need not/should not be touched. Merely lavage and drain.

b) Faecal peritonitis: the peritonitis is diffuse and the patient desperately ill. The pulse is high, blood pressure low, and there may be free gas in the peritoneal cavity and free faeculent fluid and an obvious perforation. Treatment here is not oversewing but exteriorisation of the segment with possibly a Hartmann's procedure.

112 Removal of the spleen to improve diagnostic categorisation and to reduce the irradiation dose to that area, reducing lung damage. Splenectomy also improves the haematological response to therapy and reduces the likelihood of later hypersplenism and anaemia.
Oophoropexy: the ovary is moved out of the path of the irradiation to prevent premature menopause (but the altered anatomy may make conception more difficult).
Node biopsy: in separate labelled containers place biopsies of upper (coeliac), middle (sup.mesenteric), and lower (inf. mes., or bifurcation) para-aortic lymph nodes.
Liver biopsy, usually by wedge.

113 What is the rationale for using oral cellulose (e.g. "Celevac" in diverticular disease?

114 When is surgical intervention indicated in the management of ureteric calculus?

115 What are the possible complications of a posterior dislocation of the hip?

116 What is the difference between "Maximal Acid Output" and "Peak Acid Output" of the stomach?

117 How would you treat a pyonephrosis?

113 It reduces intra-sigmoid pressure.

114 a) Complete obstruction to the kidney, or sufficient obstruction to cause progressive renal damage.

b) Repeated attacks of renal colic without advance of the stone.

c) Enlargement of the stone without it advancing down the ureter.

d) Serious uncontrolled urinary infection.

e) A stone which is obviously too large to pass.

115 a) Sciatic nerve damage.

b) Associated fractures of acetabulum, femoral shaft, or head of femur.

c) Avascular necrosis of the femoral head. The longer the delay before reduction the more likely and more severe the necrosis - which leads to degenerative arthritis.

d) Myositis ossificans.

e) Failure of reduction; if the patient presents after a long delay after dislocation closed reduction may be impossible and open reduction may be attempted.

116 M.A.O. = Quantity of Mmoles acid/litre of fluid secreted over one hour by a given stimulus.

P.A.O. = The mean of two consecutive peak 15 minute samples of gastric fluid, expressed in Mmoles/hour.

117 In all cases an attempt should be made to establish renal drainage as soon as possible. Achieve this by ureteric catheter, percutaneous needle nephrostomy or formal nephrostomy. Subsequently operate to remove the obstruction aiming for renal conservation.

118 Which is the commonest type of sarcoma of childhood?

119 In the majority of patients with diverticulosis only the sigmoid colon shows evidence of diverticula. Roughly how common are right sided diverticula?

120 You operate on a young woman for suspected appendicitis and find salpingitis. Until the results of culture of your operative swabs become available, what is your initial antibiotic treatment regimen?

121 Where might you expect to find splenunculi?

122 What is the position of the femur in posterior dislocation of the hip?

123 What are the approximate electrolyte contents of Hartmann's solution?

124 How would you manage a patient who has an asymptomatic coin lesion or pulmonary opacity on routine/mass X-ray examination?

118 Rhabdomyosarcoma (including the embryonal variety of sarcoma botryoides of female genitalia).

119 About 30% - The right side of the colon is affected exclusively in about 14% of cases.
The whole colon is affected in about 16%.

120 (Swabs from salpingitis often fail to give satisfactory bacteriological culture results.)

Metronidazole: most cases of pelvic inflammatory disease are associated with anaerobic bacteria.
(Willis et al, Lancet 1974 2 1540.)

plus

Amoxicillin or cephaloridine

121 Near the hilum of the spleen.
In the omentum.
Occasionally in the broad or ovarian ligaments.

122 Adduction, medial rotation and slight flexion.

123 Na^{+} 130, K^{+} 5, Cl^{-} 110, Lactate 30, Ca^{++} 2 (mmol/L).

124 History, examination with special reference to chest, and those systems whose tumours commonly metastasize to the lungs (which are?)

Routine investigation: F.B.C./Sputum, Culture / Cytology (T.B. fungi/ etc)
Electrolytes

Special investigations: Further/Repeat X-ray chest and screening/Tomograms/C.T. scan/Lung scan/Bronchoscopy (Brush biopsy).

If T.B. suspected Mantoux test.

Further investigations/treatment depends on results of the foregoing but may include:
Thoracotomy
Trial of anti-T.B. therapy
X.R.T.

N.B. If the lesion is obviously calcified it is probably benign and is probably either old T.B. or a hamartoma.

125 Parks has classified fistula in ano into four main types, which? *See Parks 1976 B.J.S. 63 1 - 12.*

126 In which disease is the spleen a haemopoietic organ?

127 An incompletely evacuated enema may give rise to what type of X-Ray picture of the erect abdomen?

128 What are the usual presenting symptoms of ulcerative colitis?

129 A young adult male is brought to Casualty with a probable fractured pelvis. X-Ray confirms this. You notice that he has bruising in the perineum, blood at the external urinary meatus and he cannot pass urine. Which investigations should you perform?

125 a) Intersphincteric (the fistula ramifies only in the intersphincteric plane. It is the commonest of all types and is sometimes known as the low anal type fistula. Treatment involves cutting the internal sphincter only, in contrast to the remaining three which involve cutting part of the external sphincter)

b) Transphincteric (the track passes from the intersphincteric plane through the external sphincter complex at varying levels into the ischio-rectal fossa)

c) Suprasphincteric (the track passes into the intersphincteric plane over the top of puborectalis, then downwards again through levator plate to ischio-rectal fossa and finally to the skin)

d) Extrasphincteric (the track passes from perineal skin, through the ischio-rectal fat and levator muscles into the rectum. It is outside the external sphincter complex altogether

126 B Thalassaemia Major (Cooley's anaemia)
Myelofibrosis
Chronic myeloid leukaemia
Marble bone disease.

127 Multiple fluid levels, suggesting obstruction.

128 Watery diarrhoea with mucus with or without blood.

129 After taking a history to establish whether there was any previous urinary or venereal disease, and after instituting general resuscitive measures, perform a gentle rectal examination. This occasionally reveals total disruption of the prostate from the bulbar urethra. An I.V.U. may also show bladder disruption or extravasation. Allow laparotomy or orthopaedic procedures first. Then either:

a) perform primary suprapubic catheterisation with later urethrogram and panendoscopy after 2 - 3 weeks (Mitchell);
b) perform urethrogram with aqueous dye. If normal,proceed to cystogram and,if normal,insert a fenestrated catheter. If a ruptured urethra be shown,explore and restore the anatomy with nylon sutures brought out through the perineum and perform primary urethral repair over a fenestrated catheter (Turner-Warwick).

130 Despite successful treatment of an apparently toxic dilatation of the colon by conservative means what is the usual outcome for the patient?

131 What autoclave cycles are commonly used to sterilise a surgeon's instruments?

132 Why may it be useful to measure ankle pressure in a patient with intermittent claudication before and after exercise?

133 If you choose to perform a lumbar sympathectomy via an extraperitoneal approach what structures, raised with the peritoneum must not be damaged?

134 Why should one particular incision be better than another for any particular operation? Consider the basic headings under which you would discuss this question. The word diseases can be a useful mnemonic.

135 How is a hiatus hernia demonstrated radiologically?

136 What are the large bowel complications of amoebiasis?

130 Most patients usually have to have a colectomy within one year.

131 150'C for 1 minute
132'C for 3 minutes + warm up time
121'C for 15 minutes

132 Ankle pressure measurement may indicate the severity of arterial disease and the site of a block or stenosis; the pressure may fall after exercise indicating a significant stenosis not apparent at rest.

133 The ureter and genital vessels. (On the right the sympathetic chain is partly hidden by the I.V.C. and on the left by the aorta.)

134 Damage (to nerves, muscle, fascia underlying structures)
Inconspicuous/Infection
Speed
Extensibility
Access
Strength
Exploration
Stages (i.e. staged operations, placing of colostomy etc.)

135 It may be visible in a plain chest X-ray as a gas shadow behind the heart. It will be shown by screening of a barium meal. The patient is turned to the semi-prone position on his Right side and tipped into 10 degrees trendelenburg. In the case of a true hiatus hernia barium will regurgitate into the hernia without the aid of any additional pressure. If there is no regurgitation from the hernia into the oesophagus, the hernia is usually symptomless and no treatment is necessary.

136 Colitis (which may mimic ulcerative colitis)
Haemorrhage
Granuloma formation (which may look like carcinoma)
Fibrous structure formation and/or obstruction
Perforation
Para-colic abscess or ischio-rectal abscess.

137 What methods are available for effectively lengthening a nerve, e.g. to overcome the shortening so common in soft tissue injuries with nerve damage, where scarred nerve has to be resected to obtain fresh ends for anastomosis?

138 "If it looks like a clover the trouble is over ......" Complete the rhyme.

139 How may a massive ovarian cyst be distinguished from ascites?

140 How is the carcinoid syndrome confirmed by investigation?

141 Give a list of the predisposing causes of bladder malignancy.

137 If possible always perform nerve repairs under magnification, i.e. loup or dissecting microscope. This improves the chances of obtaining a decent neurolysis and realignment of bundles in a divided nerve, facilitating 'interfascicular sutures'. Millesi has shown that in experienced hands, nerve grafting gives superior results than suturing under tension, (in which two ends of a divided nerve have to be dragged together to bridge a wide gap). Thus if the gap is not too great, mobilise the nerve ends by sharp and blunt dissection preserving the important branches. If appropriate perform a transposition (e.g. the ulnar nerve at the elbow). Anastomose the nerve ends with minimal tension, good alignment of fasciculi, adequate soft tissue and skin cover using very fine monofilament sutures. If after mobilisation of the nerve and excision of scarred nerve, the gap is too wide, use nerve or 'cable' graft or grafts. In very special circumstances such as digital replantation or brachial plexus repair, it may be advisable to shorten bone to enable direct suture.
Millesi, H., The interfascicular nerve grafting of the median and ulnar nerves. J. Bone and Joint Surg. 54-A 727-750 (1972).

138 "If it looks like a dahlia it must be a failure". (Haemorrhoidectomy)

139 This may be difficult as shifting dullness can be present in both conditions. With an ovarian cyst the swelling is more prominent in the midline with resonance in the flanks. Bimanual pelvic examination may help, as may an ultrasound scan.

140 By measurement of the 5-Hydroxyindoleacetic acid level in the urine. This can be falsely high if the patient has recently eaten bananas, or is receiving phenothiazines or reserpine.

141 a) Chemicals (Naphthylamine/Benzidine/Paraxenylamine derivatives)
b) Smoking Tryptophan derivatives
c) Calculus
d) Leucoplakia
e) Squamous metaplasia
f) Untreated ectopia vesicae
g) Schistosomiasis (Bilharzia)
h) Cystitis granulosa
i) Neurogenic bladder (increased incidence)

142 What are the indications for a Symes amputation?

143 Of what is this a description? "A small humerus (child's) appears to contain a tumour within a medullary cavity in the metaphyseal region. The cortex is perforated at one point where it has raised up the periosteum. It has an onion-peel appearance in the way new bone has formed under the periosteum. The tumour looks whitish in colour."

144 What are the common causes of abdominal distension in the newborn?

145 What is the place of systemic chemotherapy in the initial treatment of operable breast cancer?

146 What arterial disease gives rise to a 'corkscrew' or spiral pattern of vessels as seen on angiography?

147 What is the arterial supply of the bladder?

148 An I.V.U. shows reduction in size of one kidney with delayed excretion but greater concentration of contrast medium. What may this be due to?

142 There aren't many because the prosthetic replacement for a below knee amputation gives as good a functional result as that for a Symes. It is still used occasionally in wartime and in underdeveloped countries where prostheses are unavailable or unreliable or not tolerated by the patient. It may be indicated in some women where cosmesis is important, and in children who adapt to it well. It can give a sound end-bearing stump and the patient can walk without an additional prosthesis.

143 Ewing's tumour. Similar appearances can occur due to metastases from adrenal neuroblastoma.

144 Intestinal Obstruction arising in Utero.
Over-distended bladder due to urethral obstruction.
Abdominal tumours, congenital cystic kidney, or liver.
Foetal ascites - rare.
Meconium Peritonitis.

145 As yet uncertain, but the idea is becoming more fashionable. Bonadonna et al have shown statistically improved prognosis at approximately 2 years. *New England Journal of Medicine (1976) 294 405-410.*

146 Buerger's disease, and fibromuscular dysplasia of the renal arteries. The spiral pattern appears only in collaterals which open up when the main artery is occluded.

147 Inferior and superior vesical arteries from the anterior branch of the internal iliac, plus branches from the obturator and inferior gluteal, uterine or vaginal vessels in the female.

148 Unilateral renal artery stenosis.

149 What is the most common site of occurrence of squamous carcinoma of the tongue?

150 Manometry of the common bile duct shows that in a particular patient the opening pressure of the sphincter of Oddi is 30 cm of water. What is the significance of this?

151 In the first 36 hours of life a baby may vomit what - that can be considered normal?

152 When is a trans-metatarsal amputation indicated?

153 Which vessel often thromboses early in osteomyelitis of the shaft of a long bone?

154 What are the factors commonly thought to be carcinogenic in the oral cavity and oro-pharynx?

155 Which, if any, patients with acquired haemolytic anaemia are recommended to undergo splenectomy?

156 What are the alternative anatomical approaches for surgery to the common iliac arteries?

149 Lateral margin (50)%.

150 The normal opening pressure is less than 16 cm of water. Raised levels of 30 or more are associated in most cases with gallstones in the common bile duct or obstruction of its lower end *(Leader, British Medical Journal (1973)* *3 512.*

151 Swallowed amniotic fluid, vaginal secretions, blood, rarely yellow material which is due to carotene in the colostrum milk. A normal baby won't vomit bile in this period.

152 1) Following trauma - for a partially crushed foot.
2) In some cases of diabetic gangrene affecting the toes only.
3) Buerger's disease.
4) In some cases of alcoholic and nutritional neglect peripheral neuropathy. In South Africa referred to as "Vrot Voet" = Rotten foot. The U.K. equivalent might be "Tramp's foot".
5) Rarely successful salvage arterial surgery which has restored proximal circulation.

153 The nutrient artery, and thus the bone becomes dependent upon the periosteal blood supply.

154 Smoking (and tobacco and betel nut chewing)
Syphilis
Spirits
Sharp teeth
Spices

155 Those patients in whom a Chromium 51 scan with labelled red cells show that the spleen is a major site of red cell destruction, and those unresponsive to, or needing unacceptably high doses of steroids.

156 Transperitoneal (e.g. Via paramedian, midline or transverse incisions)
Extraperitoneal (e.g. Via lateral oblique incision with retroperitoneal dissection)

157 List some of the complications of peritoneal dialysis.

158 What are believed to be the causes of Metachronous tumours of the large bowel?

159 In cases of ischaemia of the foot, with which types of pathology is it reasonable to hope for primary healing from a transmetatarsal amputation?

160 What is the Boerema Button used for?

161 How common is hypospadias?

162 What type of injury does sympathetic ophthalmia follow?

163 How useful is splenectomy in a patient with acquired haemolytic anaemia and warm antibodies?

157 Surgical Procedure

Perforation of a viscus
Preperitoneal placement of catheter
Unsatisfactory drainage
Leakage of dialysis fluid

General

Pain
Haemorrhage
Infection
Pulmonary complications

Metabolic

Hypo/Hypervolaemia
Metabolic Alkalosis
Lactic Acidaemia
Hyperglycaemia
Protein/Amino Acid Loss
Disequilibrium syndrome

Late

Adhesions/Peritonitis

158 Metachronous tumours are ones appearing some time after removal of another tumour, as opposed to synchronous tumours. Many apparently metachronous tumours are, in fact, synchronous ones that were not noticed at the original operation. This emphasizes the need of thorough examination of the rest of the colon before excision of a colonic tumour. Other causes are:-

a) Recurrence of an inadequately resected tumour.

b) Implantation of tumour at an anastomosis.

c) A second primary tumour.

159 Crush or other trauma to the foot; Diabetic ischaemia; Buerger's disease.

160 Emergency surgical treatment of bleeding oesophageal varices.

161 Approximately one in every three hundred and fifty live male births (Bailey and Love).

162 A penetrating injury of the eyeball. (The untraumatised eye may be at risk from about 10 days after the injury).

163 Quite useful provided that the spleen is the major site of red cell destruction.

164 What benign neoplastic tumours occur in the larynx?

165 Describe Rammstedt's Operation.

166 You are shown a pot with a short length of bowel which has an oval shaped ulcer in it. How would you decide whether it was tuberculous or typhoidal in origin?

167 List some of the commoner anatomical anomalies of the gall-bladder and cystic duct, seen by contrast radiography.

168 Two to six weeks after laparotomy a patient presents with generalised abdominal pain, tenderness and distension but there are no specific clinical or radiological findings. (Occasionally ascites is detected or an abdominal mass). From the timing of onset of this acute abdomen what is a likely cause for this picture?

164 Squamous papilloma
Chondroma
Neurofibroma
Granular cell myoblastoma
Adenoma
Haemangioma

165 Pre-op Preparation: I.V. Fluids, often unnecessary, Achieve electrolyte balance if possible.
Empty stomach, N.G.Tube.
G.A.
Short rectus splitting incision below the Right Costal margin.
Retract Right lobe of liver out of the way.
Draw the pylorus out/into the wound.
Divide the pylorus longitudinally with Knife or cautery down to the last few fibres.
Tease the remaining muscle fibres apart with a blunt probe.
Check that you haven't perforated the mucosa of the duodenum.
Close the wound.
Resuscitate baby if necessary.
Feed the baby as soon as it has recovered.

166 Classically the long axis of the oval shape is transverse to the long axis of the bowel in T.B.; and vice versa in typhoid.

167 Phrygian cap (like a partial diverticulum of the gall-bladder).
Floating gall-bladder: mesentery predisposing to torsion.
Double gall-bladder of which one may be intrahepatic.
Absent gall-bladder - associated with high incidence of stones of common bile duct.
Low entry of cystic duct.

168 Glove powder (starch) Granulomatosis.

169 What type of controlled ventilation is usually indicated in a severe head injury?

170 In relation to the radiology of diverticular disease what is the champagne glass sign?

171 Which are the commonly used metals in orthopaedics nowadays?

172 Which patients are most at risk from exophthalmos related to thyroid disease?

173 What physical signs should you try to elicit in examining a 'short case' with a cervical rib?

174 Teratoma of the neck of the newborn may present as an obstructed labour or stillbirth. Are they Benign or Malignant?

175 What are the structures of the umbilical cord at the umbilicus?

176 To which lymph nodes does lymph from the umbilicus drain?

169 Nearly always hyperventilation. This tends to constrict cerebral vessels, thereby reducing intracranial blood volume and lowering an otherwise raised intracranial pressure. Monitoring of the latter has shown how it can rise insidiously to dangerous levels if respiration is at all embarrassed.

170 The partial filling of a diverticulum occupied by a stercolith.

171 1) Stainless steel: 18% Chromium, 10% Nickel, 3% Molybdenum, magnesium, and carbon.
2) Vitallium: an alloy of cobalt, aluminium and molybdenum.
3) Titanium.

172 Typically the middle-aged male presenting with exophthalmos before signs of hyperthyroidism appear. It may progress to ophthalmoplegia.

173 Palpate the cervical rib.
Ulnar forearm hypoaesthesia.
Wasting of small muscles of the hand (C_8 & T_1).
Coolness, cyanosis of the periphery due to damage either to the sympathetic supply or subclavian artery.

174 Most are benign.

175 Allantois (forming the urachus)
Vitello-Intestinal duct
One umbilical vein and two umbilical arteries.

176 Both axillae and both groins.

177 Is ureteric catheterisation of a patient with retroperitoneal fibrosis difficult or easy?

178 What are the main complications of fibreoptic endoscopy?

179 What are the main two types of atrial septal defect?

180 Both of the above atrial septal defects cause what kind of shunt?

181 What are the main headings under which you would discuss the management of a pathological fracture?

182 In which sort of patient should you always try and leave articular cartilage when amputating at knee level?

183 A ranula is a transparent cystic swelling in the floor of the mouth, why is it so called?

177 It is usually easy, and the catheterisation may give no hint of the fibrosis.

178 Perforation of the oesophagus or stomach.
Aspiration +/- pneumonia.
Respiratory depression from excessive intravenous sedation.
Bleeding from mucosal damage without perforation.

179 Ostium Secundum
Ostium Primum (equivalent to Atrio-Ventricular defect, 1/10th as common as secundum, but much harder to repair).

180 Left to right - but if left untreated and if severe may with increasing pulmonary resistance reverse to become a Right to Left shunt, with cyanosis (Eisenmenger syndrome).

181 Any question on 'the management' should include the following basic parts:

History
Examination (add 'with particular reference to the system Involved')
Investigations a) ward tests
b) full blood count, E.S.R., electrolytes and urea
c) special biochemical: alkaline and acid phosphatase, Bence-Jones: or serum electrophoresis etc.
d) X-Rays - plain and contrast, tomography, isotope scans

<u>Treatment</u> Medical, General and specific:
relief of pain: analgesia, splinting of the fracture if possible, radiotherapy helps in some cases.
tumour treatment: hormones for secondaries due to carcinoma of breast/thyroid cytotoxics, systemic/local adjuvant/definitive therapy.
Surgical Emergency/elective - including early internal fixation of limb fractures.

Complications
Rehabilitation/terminal care as appropriate

182 In children to maximise femoral growth.

183 Because the appearance resembles the belly of a little frog.

184 What is the platelet survival time in Idiopathic thrombocytopenic purpura, and why is splenectomy helpful?

185 Which renal or urinary calculi are not usually radio-opaque?

186 Which tissues are excised in an extended radical mastectomy?

187 Rarely a thyroid adenoma may bleed sufficiently to compress the trachea and suffocate the patient. What should be done in this situation if the diagnosis is obvious?

188 Who's sign describes pain referred to the shoulder from a ruptured spleen?

189 A hernia lying beneath the linea semilunaris between the external oblique aponeurosis and internal oblique and transversus layers is called what?

190 Have Koch's postulates been fulfilled for an infectious agent in pseudomembranous (lincomycin) colitis?

191 List the names of the different types of degrees of hypospadias.

192 What is the only symptom or sign that alone denotes probable neonatal intestinal obstruction?

193 Before making the incision for a kidney operation, what should be checked on the I.V.U. or chest/abdominal X-Ray?

194 What kind of delivery is associated with a sternomastoid tumour or torticollis?

195 Do testicular tumours ulcerate through the scrotal skin?

184 It is reduced from the normal 10 days to approximately 1-4 days. The spleen selectively destroys what are otherwise apparently normal platelets; splenectomy does not overcome the cause of the disease, but relapses are less serious and often symptomless. It is difficult to predict which patients will benefit from splenectomy, but there is no doubt that some will benefit greatly.

185 Uric acid, urate stones. (Cystine stones are usually opaque due to contained sulphur; oxalate and phosphate calculi both contain calcium).

186 Removal of the breast, both pectoral muscles, supra-clavicular and internal mammary nodes, with full clearance of the axilla.

187 One must divide the deep cervical fascia as an emergency procedure thus allowing the tumour to bulge out into the wound. The cyst containing all the blood can then be aspirated.

188 Kehr.

189 Spigelian.

190 Yes. Clostridium dificile toxin has been demonstrated in such patients faeces, the organism isolated from the gut and the disease reproduced in hamsters fed antibiotics and the clostridium. *(George et al Lancet - 1978, 1, 802)*.

191 Glandular, coronal, penile, penoscrotal and perineal.

192 Bile stained vomiting. Abdominal distension may not be present in a high intestinal obstruction and meconium may be passed even in a small bowel atresia.

193 Confirm that you are operating on the correct side. Check the lengths of R11 and R12. If these be very short, they may be difficult to palpate and the incision may be wrongly placed.

194 Breech.

195 Very seldom (unless someone has been so illadvised as to remove the primary tumour through a scrotal incision).

196 Scorer and Farrington showed in 1971 that if a testis had not descended into the scrotum by ......(what age), it will not descend on its own thereafter.

197 Why is it said to be dangerous to decompress a bladder distended by chronic urinary retention? How would you do this?

198 What abnormality is often associated with an anorectal anomaly and what investigations should be undertaken?

199 What does the left renal vein drain that the right renal vein doesn't?

200 Name some factors associated with an increased risk of breast cancer.

201 What size of endotracheal tube would you use for a one year old child?

202 What is malignant lentigo?

203 Does sepsis in the palmar aspect of the hand cause swelling locally or not?

204 What is the common site for carcinoma of the penis to develop?

205 What causes the release of enteroglucagon?

206 What serious side-effect of Practolol affecting the abdomen has been reported?

207 Why are Colles fractures ten times more common in women over the age of 60 years than in women at the age of 40?

196 One year old.

197 a) Bleeding from upper and lower urinary tract may occur.
b) Acute tubular necrosis and anuria is almost always due to inadequate fluid replacement in the face of the resultant diuresis.

If blood urea raised, decompress slowly + IV fluid.
If blood urea normal, consider postponing catheterisation until after operation to avoid infection.

198 Urological abnormalities. Every patient with an anorectal anomaly should have an I.V.P. and cystogram.

199 Left gonad and adrenal gland.

200 Known cancer in other breast.
Late first pregnancy.
Positive family history.
Bottle feeding of infants (although the protective aspect of breast feeding is disputed.

201 3.5 mm external diameter.

202 A lesion which commonly appears on the face of elderly people which starts as a perfectly smooth pigmented patch. It very slowly spreads and develops one or more foci of activity which eventually leads to tumour formation, invasion of the dermis, and endo-lymphatic spread. The time scale is often up to 10 to 15 years but can be much shorter.

203 It nearly always causes dorsal swelling first because the palmar skin is bound down by the underlying fascia that it allows minimal swelling.

204 The corona.

205 Sugars and long chain triglycerides mainly in the ilcum.

206 Sclerosing peritonitis, and this can occur several months after stopping the drug.

207 It may be largely due to age-associated osteoporosis which is marked in women. Men show nothing like as high an increased incidence with age.

208 What are the main sources of infection in pyogenic liver?

209 What are some of the commoner complications of mediastinoscopy?

210 Describe the operation of right hemicolectomy.

N.B. remember this can be either emergency or elective. Discussion of bowel prep. is a common topic in vivas. Answer this question aloud, and speak in the first person 'I would ....' rather than 'The colon is resected .... etc'.

208 a) Portal pyaemia - appendicitis, diverticulitis etc.
b) Cholangitis - secondary to malignant or calculous obstruction of the bile ducts.
c) Direct spread from contiguous pathology - cholecystitis.
d) Trauma - penetrant or blunt.
e) Infarction - embolism or sickle cell disease.
f) Cryptogenic - i.e. no obvious cause.

209 Operative:- Haemorrhage - always have packs ready and be prepared to proceed to thoracotomy.
Pneumothorax - always X-ray after the procedure.

Post-operative:- Infection
Damage to Left (possibly Right) recurrent laryngeal nerve; causing husky voice, difficulty in singing and coughing.
Keloid scarring of the wound.

210 X-match 2 units of blood. Hydrate with I.V. fluids. Nasogastric tube, catheterise under G.A. Supine position ± table tilt right side up. Prep. and drape. Right paramedian incision. Explore the abdomen for metastases. Pack small bowel off to the left. Dissect greater omentum off the right side of the transverse colon to expose the hepatic flexure, or divide a part of it to be resected with the right colon. Mobilise the ascending colon by division of lateral peritoneum in the para-colic gutter. Mobilise the terminal ileum and hepatic flexure. Bring the colon and terminal ileum out of the abdomen by blunt dissection, carefully avoiding damage to duodenum, ureter, gonadal vessels. Decide the optimal sites of resection, remove at least four inches of ileum because of doubtful blood supply. Hold the bowel up against the light to see the major vessels. Try to retain at least one division of the middle colic artery to provide nutrition to the colonic side of the anastomosis. Clamp-tie-divide the mesentery progressively dividing the ileo-colic, right colic and marginal vessels. Pack off the bowel to reduce spill and then clamp it. Transect the bowel and perform an anastomosis. This can be end to end, side to side, end to side or vice versa, according to the relative luminal size and individual preference. Most surgeons prefer a two layer closure. Close the gap in the mesentery to prevent internal hernia. Remove packs. Change gloves. Close the abdomen in layers. Drainage is advisable. Discuss postoperative care, physiotherapy, complications and their management.

211 Operations to correct 'knock-knee' in a case of rickets may include stapling or osteotomy - what should be excluded first before embarking on operation?

212 Categorise the main indications for tracheostomy.

213 What criteria are used to assess whether a Dormia basket could be used to extract a ureteric stone?

214 What are the two main types of primary carcinoma occurring in the liver?

215 What special radiological investigations should be done in a patient prior to an abdomino-perineal excision of the rectum?

216 In which direction does the trachea run, below the point at which a tracheostomy is performed?

217 What is the most frequent complication of a child's colostomy and how is it treated?

218 What is the normal blood volume per kg. of a neonate?

211 Renal rickets. Operation can provoke an uraemic crisis.

212

Central	Efferent N	Neuromuscular Jnctn.
Coma	Polio	Muscle relaxants
C.V.A.	Polyneuritis	Myasthenia
Head Injury	Cervical cord lesion	

Muscles of Resp.	Airway
Tetanus Trauma	Anything obstructing airways e.g. haemorrhage, foreign body, carcinoma, inflammation. Planned procedure, e.g. with laryngectomy. Endotracheal tube in situ too long.

213 The Dormia basket may be used in the following circumstances:-

a) A small stone 6 mm or less in smallest diameter.
b) Stone must lie close to the bladder below the level of the iliac spines.
c) A reasonable trial of conservative management must have failed.
d) The ureter must be virgin (i.e. no previous operation, no stricture below the stone, and no infection).
e) A skilled operator with facilities for fluoroscopic control must be available.

214 Liver cell carcinoma (hepato-cellular carcinoma) Intra-hepatic bile duct carcinoma (cholangiocellular carcinoma).

215 A barium enema to exclude synchronous tumours elsewhere in the colon, and many surgeons also ask for an I.V.U. to exclude ureteric involvement by the tumour, and a liver scan.

216 It passes down and posteriorly. Thus a bronchoscopy is possible though not necessarily easy through a tracheostomy.

217 Prolapse of the colostomy is very common in children. It can usually be reduced by firm, steady manual compression with either sedation or an anaesthetic.

218 Approximately 85 ml/kg.

219 What are the main hazards of removing a very large tumour from the abdomen. (i.e. an ovarian cyst containing ten litres of fluid?

220 What are the indications for fibrinolytic therapy?

221 Why is biopsy of the pancreas in suspected carcinoma considered difficult or dangerous?

222 What does Ortolani's test detect?

223 When is block dissection of the neck indicated?

224 What are the causes of extra-dural abscesses?

225 Describe some of the typical peri-anal lesions of Crohn's disease.

219 Pre and post operative labile cardiovascular state with possible hypotension, or cardiac failure from sudden increase in venous return. Respiratory embarrassment from lack of splintage of the diaphragm with weak abdominal musculature. Rapid intestinal distension may also complicate the picture.

220 Massive pulmonary embolism.
Extensive D.V.T. +/- smaller pulmonary embolism.
Major vein or artery thrombosis.
(Streptokinase is now usually given intravenously and not intra-arterially).

221 Haemorrhage may be difficult to control.
Fistula formation.
Uncertainty about taking a representative specimen.
Difficult interpretation on frozen section.
N.B. Needle biopsy is becoming more popular than open biopsy and reduces the above problems.

222 Congenital dislocation of the hips in a baby. Lateral rotation and abduction of the flexed hip imparts a 'clunk' to the thumb resting on the femoral head.

223 Palpable lymph nodes involved by metastatic disease which have either failed to respond to radiotherapy or thought to be best treated surgically from the outset. Prophylactic block dissection of the neck without clinically involved nodes is still a controversial procedure.

224 Osteomyelitis of the skull is the primary pathology. It is usually secondary to frontal sinusitis or otitis media/mastoiditis. However it can follow direct infection from a compound fracture, extension from a scalp cellulitis or, rarely, blood spread of a disseminated infection.

225 Oedema of the skin with red-dusky cyanotic tinge. Indolent looking painless fissures with adjacent skin tags. Perianal or ischio-rectal abscesses. Fistulae low and high. Painless indolent ulcers.

226 What histological changes may be found after 'simple' cerebral concussion?

227 What are the common tests of adrenal activity?

228 Through which artery or arteries do the coeliac and superior mesenteric arteries anastomose?

229 If you were asked to discuss the management of a patient with a chronically ischaemic limb, part of which had become gangrenous, it would be wise to divide up the question in relation to the different basic pathologies. How might you do this?

230 What is believed to be the common cause of thrombosis of the superior mesenteric artery?

231 Scalene node biopsy is very useful for detecting extra-thoracic lymphatic spread of lung cancer, but what investigation has largely superseded this except for palpably enlarged nodes?

232 Which type of carcinoma most commonly affects the submandibular gland?

233 How soon after the onset of acute ischaemia of a leg due to embolism should you perform an embolectomy?

226 Capillary haemorrhages, clustering of microglial cells, the phagocytic response to trauma, anoxic cell changes, chromatolysis in the brain stem.

The concept that 'simple' concussion is not associated with organic brain damage has been abandoned.

227 Urinary 17 ketogenic steroids and 17 hydroxycortico-steroids.
Plasm cortisol levels at midnight and noon.
A.C.T.H. stimulation test.
Cortisol suppression test.

228 The superior and inferior pancreatico-duodenal arteries. (The coeliac supplies the foregut and the superior mesenteric is the artery of the midgut).

229 There are several alternative classifications, and the one you choose is up to you. Here are two:-

a) Atheroma
b) Raynaud's
c) Buerger's
d) Ergotamine poisoning

a) Arterial
1. Large vessel (atheroma)
2. Medium vessel (atheroma, embolic)
3. Small vessel (vasculitis, diabetic, embolic)

b) Venous
c) Combined arterial and venous

230 Atheroma of the first 2-3 cm of the artery.

231 Mediastinoscopy. (Introduced in 1959, allowing inspection of both sides of the mediastinum and lymph node biopsy from nodes much closer to the probable carcinoma.)

232 Adenoid cystic carcinoma. This has a predilection for spreading along nerve sheaths and the lingual nerve may thus have to be sacrificed.

233 As soon as possible. After 8 hours the chances of obtaining a viable limb decrease sharply.

234 How do you assess and record muscle power?

235 At laparotomy for large bowel obstruction in an otherwise fit 55 year old man you find a moderate degree of obstruction, a resectable sigmoid carcinoma and multiple large hepatic secondaries. How would you proceed?

236 What is the commonest form of dislocation of the elbow?

237 1. What is the treatment of carcinoma of the tonsil?
2. What is the overall five year survival?

238 Why should you inform the anaesthetist that a patient is receiving streptomycin, neomycin or gentamicin?

239 Following neurotmesis how fast can you expect the axons to grow after careful nerve suture?

240 Why may stripping of the long saphenous vein frequently fail to cure stasis ulcers?

234 0.....Total paralysis
1.....Barely detectable contraction
2.....Insufficient to overcome gravity
3.....Just sufficient to overcome gravity
4.....Stronger than 3 but less than full power
5.....Normal

235 This is controversial. The standard answer is either a three stage procedure (proximal colostomy now, interval sigmoid resection, later colostomy closure), or a two stage procedure (sigmoid resection with colostomy and then later closure of colostomy). Many surgeons consider that the hepatic secondaries indicate a limited prognosis and justify a one stage operation to prevent long periods of hospitalisation for the patient. However, a one stage procedure of resection and primary anastomosis should only be done by an experienced surgeon, when the anastomosis looks viable and the obstruction not too advanced.

236 Lateral and posterior. Thus, achieve reduction by medial pulsion and slight traction. After reduction check the medial epicondyle radiologically for fracture and confirm the integrity of the nerves and arteries - radial, median and ulnar nerves and brachial artery (these should have been checked before attempting the reduction).

237 1. Primary DXT with follow-up radical neck dissection if necessary OR combined therapy of XRT (approx. 3000 Rads) followed, 10 days later, by a 'commando' operation.

2. Approximately 25% five year survival.

238 Like other aminoglycosides, these drugs have some neuromuscular blocking properties.

239 About 1 - 1.5 mm per day although experimentally they have been found to grow as much as 4 mm per day.

240 The long saphenous vein usually does not communicate with the deep axial vessels by those perforators whose incompetence causes the ulceration.

241 Describe the basic steps involved in an abdominal hysterectomy. This occasionally has to be done by general surgeons incidental to other procedures.

242 What are some of the major problems of stilboestrol therapy in prostatic cancer?

243 In the case of a medial meniscus tear which is particularly painful - internal or external rotation of the leg on the thigh?

244 What is currently the common method of treatment of sub-clinoid aneurysms?

245 What are the symptoms and signs of a ruptured urethra in the male?

241 Abdominal hysterectomy. With the patient in the Trendelenberg position pack intestines out of the pelvis. Use strong Kochers forceps and always keep close to the uterus. Double clamp the round ligament and the ovarian pedicle close to the uterus so the points are in the avascular area above the uterine vessels, on each side. Divide the pedicles and double ligate using 1 chromic catgut. Use the medial forceps for traction on the uterus. Divide the utero-vesical fold of peritoneum transversely close to the uterus and sweep the bladder down off lower uterus and cervix. Place straight Kochers transversely across the uterine vessels at the level of utero-cervical junction, divide the artery medial to the forceps. Incise the cervico-vesical fascia transversely across anterior cervix and sweep bladder on to the longitudinal fibres of the vagina. Place angled Kochers across the vaginal angles - above the bladder and ureters and incise into the vagina medial to the forceps. Divide the vagina anteriorly and posteriorly close to the cervix and remove the uterus. Double ligate each uterine pedicle, transfixing the inferior border of the pedicle, using 1 chromic catgut. The vaginal angles are similarly sutured once only using 1 chromic catgut. The vaginal vault is repaired with continuous suture of 0 Dexon or catgut. The pelvic peritoneum is repaired, leaving the pedicles extraperitoneal with 0 catgut. The abdominal wall is closed in layers and a rectus sheath vacuum drain used if the incision is transverse.

242 Resistent cancer.
Fluid retention (especially dangerous with heart disease).
Thromboembolism.
Embarrassing gynaecomastia.
Impotence.
Liver damage with higher doses.

243 External rotation.

244 Ligation of the common carotid artery.

245 Pain, perineal haematoma, blood at the external urinary meatus, and urinary retention.

246 What is the disadvantage of the portex tracheostomy tube compared to the silver tube?

247 Both anaplastic and papillary carcinoma of the thyroid infiltrate local lymph nodes. What are the differences in the clinical characteristics of these infiltrated nodes?

248 List some preventative factors associated with a lower incidence of wound infection.

249 If you were fated to develop rectal cancer in which part of the rectum might you hope that it would develop?

250 What does a mulberry urinary stone consist of?

251 In whom and where are you most likely to find an ependymoma?

246 It does not have an inner tube which can be removed for clearing the airway. It does not incorporate a fenestration in the shoulder nor an expiratory valve which allows the expiratory tide to pass through the larynx enabling the patient to speak.

247 Papillary carcinoma is associated with discrete rubbery or cystic nodes which generally remain static for long periods - i.e. several months; anaplastic carcinoma leads to firmer nodes which become rapidly fixed to local structures.

248 a) Minimal in-patient stay.
b) Elimination of co-existent infection.
c) Avoidance of abrasions/cuts in skin shaving. Use of depilatory agents in preference to shaving.
d) Adequate skin cleansing/preparation at the operation site.
e) Laminar air flow over the operating table (controversial).
f) Pre-operative prophylactic systemic antibiotics (controversial).
g) Operative - Minimal operating time
Strict asepsis
Meticulous haemostasis
Avoidance of wound drains in clean wounds
Delayed primary closure of contaminated wounds
Local antibiotics in wounds before closure (controversial, but widely accepted *Gilmore and Sanderson 1975 BJS 62, 792-799)*.

249 In the upper third. The prognosis is better here, possibly because the peritoneum prevents early spread. Also an anterior resection will almost certainly be possible even if you are fat!

250 Mainly calcium oxalate (it may have another nidus). It is sharp, hard, often symptomatic when small and may cause local bleeding thus staining the stone.

251 In the fourth ventricle of a child.

252 What are the indications for surgery in a blow-out fracture of the orbit?

253 Where is the foramen of Morgagni?

254 Which type of hyperthyroid patient is best treated by long term anti-thyroid medication such as carbimazole?

255 What may be the cause of G.I.T. bleeding in a severely burned patient.

256 What is the meaning of the words prevalence and incidence?

257 How would you assess whether a hand infection demands incision and drainage?

258 Where is a post intubation granuloma found?

259 Weakness of the extensor hallucis longus in a case of possible prolapsed intervertebral disc places the lesion where?

252 a) Incarceration of orbital contents into the fracture with consequent globe retraction and raised intra-ocular pressure on upward gaze.
b) A fracture with a large herniation of tissue into the antrum.
c) Enophthalmos of 3 mm or more.
d) Diplopia not resolving significantly within the first ten days after the injury.

253 It is a congenital defect between the sternal and costal attachments of the diaphragm. It is the site of one type of diaphragmatic hernia.

254 Young females. N.B. Start with a high dose of carbimazole plus small replacement dose of thyroxine or diatroxine (90% T_4 + 10% T_3) for six months and then start to reduce the dose.

255 Curling's ulcer. This carries a high mortality: is associated with, but not necessarily caused by, high gastrin and glucagon levels.
(Orton et al B.M.J. (1975) 2 170-172.)

256 Prevalence covers all cases detected at a particular time in a given population, whereas incidence implies the number of cases occurring over a specified period of time in a given population.

257 A useful guideline is that if the patient's pain which is obviously due to infection prevents him from sleeping, the hand sepsis should be decompressed by incision and drainage.

258 On the vocal process of the arytenoid cartilage which forms the posterior ¼ of the vocal cord. (it is due to friction or pressure ischaemia by the tube causing infection.)

259 Usually the disc between L.4 and L.5 pressing on the L.5 nerve root.

260 Give a very brief classification of lung cysts.

261 Which serious complication of resection for bronchial carcinoma may be more frequent if pre-operative radiotherapy is used?

262 Where do metastases of an anterior 2/3 tongue carcinoma drain to?

263 Where does gastric atrophy occur in the stomach in patients with pernicious anaemia?

264 Is the atrophy reversible?

265 Of what is a smooth staghorn calculus composed?

266 You are given a 'short case' with ulceration of the tongue. What is the differential diagnosis that must flash through your mind as you examine the patient?

267 How much ileum is cleared of mesentery in fashioning an ileostomy?

268 Is surgery ever indicated in the treatment of bacterial endocarditis?

269 What are the radiological features of gastric atrophy?

260 Epithelial. (Developmental, large/small, single/multiple, lined by epithelium with traces of cartilage, muscle, glands.)
Emphysematous
Parasitic (hydatid for example)
Pseudocysts (cavities resembling cysts).

261 Broncho-pleural fistula. Rare after lobectomy, less rare after pneumonectomy.

262 From tongue tip to submental nodes, then to jugulo-omohyoid and then to lower deep cervical nodes. The further back the lesion on the tongue, the higher the group of cervical nodes involved. (The lymphatics follow the primitive embryological folds.)

263 In the fundus and body but not the antrum.

264 No. Irreversible despite long continued Vit. B_{12} injection.

265 Phosphates.

266 Carcinoma, gumma, T.B., 'simple ulcer'.

267 About 7.5 cm.

268 Yes. Surgery has an important place in the infective stage when there is intractable heart failure.
English and Ross, B.M.J. 1972 4 598-602.

269 The stomach is usually small, with tubular outline and loss of the usual folds on the greater curve and in the fundus. The antral folds are normal, but the folds in the body are thin and crenated like tissue paper. The duodenal cap is normal.

270 What is the cause of hydrocele in infancy and childhood?

271 What is the correct order of X-ray investigation of a possible cervical spine injury?

272 Which umbilical herniae in infants and children should be repaired?

273 You are shown a 'pot' which has a kidney and an adrenal gland in it. You are told that it came from a woman of fifty years of age. You note that in the adrenal cortex there is a tiny tumour. You also notice that the kidney is shrivelled and scarred especially around the pelvis of the kidney. What did this woman suffer from?

274 Which adult patients in particular are likely to damage a fibre-optic endoscope through failure to respond to the normal sedating dose of diazepam, and for whom therefore a general anaesthetic is probably indicated?

275 Ectopic A.C.T.H. production is often associated with what type of acid base disturbance?

276 At similar clinical stages, which is more sinister - melanotic or amelanotic melanoma?

277 A skull X-ray of a child or adolescent which shows an enlarged pituitary fossa, and calcification in that region, is likely to be due to what pathology?

270 Persistence of a communication between the peritoneum and the tunica vaginalis, allowing fluid from the peritoneal cavity to collect in the tunica vaginalis. Secondary hydroceles are rare, and idiopathic type not seen.

271 a) Before the neck is moved plain A/P and lateral views including C_7 if possible are obtained.

b) If there is no obvious change, better views can be taken of the same and then: Open mouth views of the odontoid process. If mandibular fracture or trismus prevent the latter, tomograms may be necessary.
c) If there is no odontoid fracture then it is safe to ask for flexion and extension and lateral flexion views.

272 a) Those which fail to decrease in size and close by school age. (Generally those whose defect is more than 1.5 cm diameter at the neck of the hernia.)

b) Rare cases causing pain or becoming incarcerated.

273 Conn's syndrome. Hypertension, hypokalaemia, low renin level, secondary pyelonephritis.

274 Young adult alcoholics, drug addicts or epileptics.

275 Hypokalaemic alkalosis. (Potassium level less than 3 mmol/l and bicarbonate over 30 mmol/l.)

276 Amelanotic.

277 Craniopharygioma. (It often presents with visual loss, raised I.C.P. and failure to grow and mature sexually.)

278 List the benign neoplasms of the breast.

279 How should you describe a fracture if asked to comment on an X-ray depicting one?

280 What is the end result of untreated posterior compartment syndrome?

281 What is the treatment?

282 What modified type of block dissection of the neck may be considered for a patient with a carcinoma of floor of mouth (anteriorly), where no nodes are palpable?

283 You are asked to write an essay on the use of isotopes in surgery - how might you divide the subject up?

284 What is the treatment of chylothorax?

278 Epithelial: Intraduct papilloma
Pure adenoma

Conn. Tissue: Neurofibroma
Lipoma

Mixed: Fibroadenoma (Peri- and intra-canalicular)
Papillary cystadenoma

279 Before committing yourself it is wise to ask for other contemporaneous views, and if there is any possibility of the lucent line you see being an epiphysis, ask to see an X-ray of the other side. Nevertheless the correct answer must include the following in regard to the fracture:-

Situation, line of fracture i.e. transverse/spiral/oblique/comminuted, and displacement i.e. shift/tilt/twist. Look for periosteal reaction and callus formation; both indicate an older healing fracture; state of soft tissues, whether simple or compound fracture.

280 Claw toes, inability to extend the toes, anaesthesia in the distribution of the posterior tibial nerve in toes and foot.

281 Surgical decompression - splitting of the whole length of fascia enclosing the compartment with delayed primary suture or grafting.

282 A bilateral supra-hyoid block dissection

283 Diagnostic: In vitro - Radioimmunoassay
In vivo - Scanning of organs, limbs etc.

Therapeutic: Destruction of tissue selectively.

284 Initially conservative, low fat diet, wait and watch. If after 2 weeks leakage continues then operate to ligate the duct.

285 What is the radiological sign of a duodenal obstruction in the neonate?

286 What mechanical and chemical means are believed to reduce the incidence of post-operative D.V.T.?

287 What methods are available for sterilising RE9 heat sensitive apparatus?

288 If asked to discuss or compare the qualities of two different suture materials, what should your answer include?

289 At what level do you amputate the femur for a Stokes-Gritti amputation?

290 Which foramen does the middle meningeal artery traverse?

291 What simple bed-side test will indicate whether a patient has a recurrent laryngeal nerve palsy or paresis?

285 The double bubble i.e. air/fluid level in a dilated stomach and air/fluid level in a dilated duodenum.

286 Mechanical: Static graduated leg compression
Passive leg exercise
Electrical stimulation of calf muscle
Intermittent pneumatic compression of legs

Chemical: Intravenous dextran
Warfarin
Subcutaneous heparin
Intra-venous lignocaine

Combined methods: Oxyphenbutazone + static compression
Subcutaneous heparin + intermittent compression
Aspirin + dipyridamole.

287 a) Ethylene oxide: reliable under microbiological control or in commercial use.
b) Gamma irradiation: commercial use.
c) Low temperature steam: ability controversial (spores formalin autoclave in doubt)
d) Buffered gluteraldehyde: independent assessment suggests spores only killed by freshly prepared solutions.
e) Methanol-hypochlorite: experimental.

288 a) The degree of inflammatory response.
b) The behaviour of the suture material in the presence of infection.
c) The durability of the material.
d) Its handling abilities, and strength.
e) Price.

289 At the level of the adductor tubercle.

290 Foramen spinosum.

291 Either ask the patient to give a good cough (which requires closure of the glottis) or ask him to sing which he will find difficult if he has one nerve paralysed.

292 What is the treatment of osteochondritis dissecans?

293 A newborn baby regurgitates all its first and subsequent feeds and foamy saliva pours from its mouth and nostrils. You suspect oesophageal atresia. How far would you expect a nasal catheter to pass in such a case? What is the commonest form of oesophageal atresia?

294 Why do relatively few surgeons delegate the use of the Dormia basket to junior staff?

295 Where would you expect to locate the tear in a spontaneous rupture of the oesophagus?

296 What is the commonest presenting symptom of renal tuberculosis?

297 List some of the possible space-occupying lesions of the anterior mediastinum.

298 Which blood group antibodies have particular relevance to open heart surgery?

299 What serious complication may occur to the contra-lateral lung in diaphragmatic hernia?

292 For minimal or mild symptoms - stop sport.
For severe symptoms or locking of a joint - explore the joint, remove loose fragments, curette the crater(s). If the fragment is undisplaced try drilling the fragment to stimulate blood supply. The pinning of fragments which have separated is controversial.

293 11 cm from the nostril. The commonest form of oesophageal atresia (85%) shows a blind ended upper oesophagus, the lower oesophagus entering the trachea close to the bifurcation.

294 a) It cannot be used under direct vision (although X-ray fluoroscopy is very helpful) and has been known to cause serious large tears in the ureter.
b) The basket can become stuck requiring open operation for its own removal.
c) Many consider that the procedure's dangers are too great for such delegation.

295 It is usually 1 - 4 cm long, longitudinal, in the left posterior wall of the extreme lower end of the oesophagus. It usually fills the mediastinum not peritoneal cavity with air, and after six or more hours the pleura gives way and fluid enters the pleural cavity.

296 Day and night urinary frequency (accompanied by sterile pyuria).

297 Retro-sternal goitre
Thymic cysts or tumours
Persistently enlarged thymus
Teratoma
Pleuro-pericardial cyst.

298 Those acting at low temperature. The blood for this type of surgery is screened pre-operatively for low temperature antibodies (e.g. anti I and anti P).

299 Pneumothorax occurs in approximately 20%.

300 What is the common site for congenital valves of the urethra?

301 Do you push or pull a celestin tube down towards the stomach to overcome oesophageal narrowing?

302 What are the advantages of a renogram over an I.V.U. in determining kidney function?

303 How important is hiatus hernia as a cause of gastro-intestinal bleeding?

304 What type of cutaneous tumour may be given the following possible macroscopic descriptions:- nodular, cystic, cicatrising, superficial multicentric, ulcerated?

305 In what circumstances may a urinary diversion be necessary?

306 After how much blood loss should a baby or infant be transfused at operation?

300 Valves are circumferentially arranged arising at the lower margin of the verumontanum and extending obliquely around the urethra to meet at a lower level on the anterior urethral wall. Between them the urethral lumen is a narrow slit.

301 The celestin tube is gently pulled down rather than blindly pushed as with a Souttar tube.

302 A renogram is quantitative if subtraction techniques are used. Iodine sensitivity is unimportant, and X-irradiation is one hundreth of the dose used in I.V.U., both may be done as an emergency, and a renogram may be helpful in uraemia.

303 Hiatus hernia itself is not often a cause of bleeding as used to be commonly said; when bleeding is related it is usually due to ulcers at the level of the hernia or, more commonly, to gastro-oesophageal reflux and resultant oesophagitis.

304 Basal cell carcinoma.

305 Carcinoma of the bladder Total cystectomy for such conditions as confluent superficial transitional cell carcinoma which fails to respond to cystodiathermy, epodyl, or hydrodistension; well differentiated supratrigonal tumour given pre-operative radiotherapy.
Small irritant bladder Interstitial cystitis, post-irradiation cystitis.
Female incontinence When intractable. Sphincter disturbance. Neurogenic bladder.
Congenital anomalies Ectopia vesicae etc.

306 If the blood loss is 10% or more of the blood volume, then a transfusion should be given: e.g. 2 kg. neonate blood volume 2 x 85 = 170 ml., therefore, if the blood loss is 17 ml. or above, transfuse.

307 What X-ray studies are needed in a kidney donor prior to surgery?

308 Post gastrectomy syndromes are often divided into two types a) post cibal b) nutritional. What are the important features of each type?

309 What volume of contrast medium do you need to inject up a retrograde ureteric catheter to outline the pelvis of a normal sized kidney?

310 What are the causes of Cushing's syndrome?

311 What is the five year survival of patients with a carcinoma of the anterior 2/3 of the tongue?

312 Most trials of Wilm's tumour therapy quote a ....year survival of 30-50% in all cases.

313 After excision of a skin tumour in what circumstances is it often preferable to close the defect with a flap rather than a free skin graft?

314 What proportion of kidneys have more than one arterial supply?

307 Plain X-rays of abdomen and chest, an I.V.U. and preferably an aortogram to identify anomalous arteries which might make the kidney unsuitable for transplantation.

308 Post Cibal: Early dumping
Late hypoglycaemia
Bilious vomiting

Nutritional: Small stomach - reduced intake - weight loss
Steatorrhoea) or gross malabsorption
Diarrhoea)
Fe. deficiency anaemia
Megaloblastic anaemia: B_{12} deficiency
Calcium deficiency

309 About 2-4 ml; retrogrades are less frequently needed nowadays with better I.V.U's, and bulb ureterograms are usually more useful for outlining upper tract problems.

310 a) Iatrogenic - steroid and A.C.T.H. administration.
b) Excess A.C.T.H. secretion by the pituitary.
c) Adrenocortical adenoma or carcinoma.
d) 'Ectopic A.C.T.H.' secretion, e.g. by tumours of bronchus.

311 About 60%

312 Two year survival is the relevant period.

313 a) When the anatomy demands it, e.g. full thickness eyelid loss.
b) When a split skin graft is likely to fail: e.g. in the presence of a salivary fistula, on bare bone, over synovium, etc.
c) When radiotherapy may be needed afterwards.

314 About 25%.

315 How are renal tumours staged?

316 Which conditions affecting the penis may be precancerous?

317 What factors determine the prognosis of a patient with a nephroblastoma?

318 What are the main types of calcaneal fracture?

319 What is the incidence and sex ratio of congenital pyloric stenosis?

320 What abnormality of the gut may be found in association with congenital diaphragmatic hernia?

321 What is the eponym for the congenital posterolateral diaphragmatic hernia? (N.B. This one generally presents in the first few days of life as a severe respiratory emergency, but may present in childhood or adulthood.)

322 What is the system by which Mr. Graham Apley recommends that a joint should be examined - and seen to be examined?

323 What is the cutaneous distribution of the C.1 spinal nerve?

315 There are many methods. One simple one is:
i) Limited to renal capsule.
ii) Invasion of pedicle and renal fat.
iii) Regional nodes involved.
iv) Demonstrable distant metastases.
(Hocres and Kadesky 1958 J. Urol. <u>*79*</u> *196.)*

316 a) Leukoplakia.
b) Long standing papilloma.
c) Long standing phimosis.
d) Paget's disease of the penis (erythroplasia of Queryat).

317 The age of the patient.
The grade of, or maturity of the tumour histologically.
The volume of the tumour removed. Empirically much worse over 550 ml.
Evidence of spread at the time of surgery.

318 Chip, split and crush fractures. It is important to note whether the integrity of the subtalar joint has been destroyed.

319 0.3% of all live births, 5 males, 1 female (50% are first born children).

320 Malrotation of the mid-gut. An abdominal approach to the repair of the hernia enables correction of the malrotation.

321 Hernia of Bochdalek.

322 Look: At the patient as a whole. Locally at the joint: skin, shape, position, shortening.
Feel: Skin, soft tissues, bones.
Move: Range, muscles, function.
X-ray.

323 It doesn't have one, only muscular and deep sensory.

324 What skin tumour does this description fit:-
'It probably arises in the hair matrix of pilo-sebaceous follicles. It forms a hard smooth rounded lump under the skin and can arise anywhere, in either sex, at any time. In spite of its name only a quarter of them show calcification. Such calcification may appear as a whitish nodule within the lump. Microscopically, the epithelium produces an abnormally large amount of keratin to which there may be a foreign body reaction.'

325 What happens to the fibrinogen level in acute pancreatitis?

326 Jones in 1978 put forward criteria for selecting suitable patients for ileorectal anastomosis rather than permanent ileostomy in the treatment of ulcerative colitis. *B.M.J. 1978 1 1459-1463)* What are these criteria?

327 In the leg, what are the commonest two causes of the 'posterior compartment syndrome'?

328 What is the usual major complication associated with a horseshoe kidney? How would you treat it?

329 Is a male or female infant more likely to develop a strangulated inguinal hernia?

330 The following histological description of soft tissue swelling is of what?
'A nodule with extensive central area of necrotic collagen which is surrounded by a zone of erectly orientated fibroblasts, which forms a palisade around it. In the periphery there is an infiltration of lymphocytes, plasma cells and macrophages.'

331 What is Caffey's disease?

324 'Calcifying epithelioma of Malherbe'. (N.B. Quite benign.)

325 It is usually raised at the end of the first week returning to normal by the third week after the start of the attack.

326 Patients who could be offered the choice between excision or retention of the rectum should have a macroscopically normal looking anal canal and rectum, capable of distension. Minimal inflammatory changes did not exclude patients if under the age of 25 years. If a colectomy must be done urgently or as an emergency it is quite acceptable to leave the rectum (unless rectal haemorrhage is a major problem) thereby postponing any decision.

327 Fractured tibia, severe deep burns, especially circumferential.

328 Hydronephrosis due to a high origin of the ureter from the renal pelvis. Treat by pyeloplasty avoiding any aberrant renal vessels.

329 Female. (Ratio 5 females to 1 male.)

330 A rheumatoid nodule.

331 Infantile cortical hyperostosis. Infants develop mandibular and/or long bone swellings which may be tender, and associated with fever. Spontaneous recovery is the rule.

332 Enumerate some of the complications of a subphrenic abscess.

333 When should the diathermy snare not be used to remove a sessile polyp seen through the sigmoidoscope?

334 How is the adequacy of theatre ventilation now assessed?

335 After removal of a stone in a pyelo-ureterolithotomy, what else should be done before closing the incision?

336 Squamous stratified epithelium on the surface of lymphoid tissue is histological identification of what?

337 Liver damage and cholangitis, in a Chinese person may present as a surgical case with biliary obstruction, and caused by an infestation with what?

338 The stellate ganglion overlies what bony structure?

332 General: Septicaemia
Cachexia

C.N.S.: Cerebral abscess
Meningitis

Thoracic: Pleural effusion
Diaphragmatic perforation
Empyema
Pyopneumothorax
Bronchopneumonia
Bronchial fistula (rare)
Pericarditis
Mediastinitis
Lung abscess (rare)

Abdominal: Hepatic abscess
Spread locally
General peritonitis ± later loculation, e.g. as pelvic abscess
Wound dehiscence
Perforation of the abscess into other viscera

333 Sessile polyps are difficult to snare anyway, and certainly this should not be attempted when they lie above the peritoneal reflection.

334 a) By air counts of bacteria or particles in the room using a slit-sampler or using settle plates.
b) By aeronometer checks over doorways.

335 In the case of a pyelolithotomy, perform on-table X-ray to confirm complete removal of the stone(s). Check for other stones or stricture lower down the ureter by simple bouginage.

336 Tonsil.(N.B. The tonsil is also distinguished by the fact that it consists of lymphoid follicles only, without a medulla and no subcapsular lymph space.)

337 Clonorchis sinensis.

338 The transverse process of C.7., and the neck of the first rib.

339 Give a brief description of the important features of a de Quervain's thyroiditis.

340 What are some of the presenting features of a choledochal cyst?

341 What is the organism commonly associated with a fulminant parotitis?

342 What is the probable cause of bilateral nipple discharge of green toothpaste-like material in a multiparous woman in her thirties?

343 What are the three common solid tumours of children?

344 Where is the fracture line in a Le Fort I fracture?

345 How does nephroblastoma spread?

346 How is the incidence of malignancy in large bowel adenomatous polyps related to size?

347 What serum factor is often increased in renal cell carcinoma?

339 A self-limiting goitre of viral aetiology, presenting as either an asymptomatic, irregular, hard, enlargement of one or both lobes, or a painful tender enlargement of acute onset with fever, malaise and possible hyperthyroidism. The E.S.R. is raised but I^{131} uptake low, and no thyroid antibodies are detectable.
It usually responds rapidly to prednisone 10-20 mg per day for a week, the dose tailing off according to response (and an early sign is a rapid drop in the E.S.R.).

340 Jaundice in the newborn.
Pain)
Mass) in the child or adult.
Jaundice)
It may just present as a painful or painless obscure hypochondrial mass or it may lead to biliary cirrhosis.

341 Staphylococcus aureus.

342 Almost certainly duct ectasia.

343 Neuroblastoma, Wilm's, Rhabdomyosarcoma.

344 It passes across the base of the maxillary antrum on either side and across the floor of the nose through the septum. Thus it is a maxillary fracture only.

345 Via blood stream most importantly, to lungs, vertebrae, liver. Local spread also important, but surprisingly the para-aortic glands although often enlarged are seldom involved.

346 Invasive carcinoma is found in approx.:-
45% if the polyp exceeds 2 cm diameter
9% if the polyp is between 1-2 cm diameter
1% if the polyp is less than 1 cm diameter
(Muto, Bussey, Morson, Cancer (1975) 36 2251)

347 Haptoglobin. Thus the serum globulin concentration rises.

348 How is a vesico-vaginal fistula usually repaired?

349 What investigation should be carried out prior to any thyroid operation both for medico-legal purposes and to establish a baseline for management of the postoperative patient?

350 Enumerate and distinguish between the various descriptions used in discussing the undescended testicle.

351 What is a sliding inguinal hernia?

352 Which patients with ulcerative colitis are at particular risk of developing carcinoma?

353 When is nephrolithotomy rather than pyelolithotomy indicated? Are they ever both performed together?

354 How much of what substance is given to reverse the action of phenindione?

348 The underlying cause must first be sought and treated appropriately (i.e. neoplasm, tuberculosis, irradiation damage). A vaginal approach may be used, the edges are freshened, and through and through sutures used to close the fistula. The bladder should be drained for 14 days at least to prevent any tension from bladder distension during wound healing. Some surgeons prefer to approach these fistulae from above perhaps utilising omentum.

349 Indirect laryngoscopy. Up to 3% of the population have an asymptomatic partial or complete vocal cord palsy.

350 'Undescended testicle' is a vague term within the whole field of imperfect descent. This may be incomplete = normal or abnormal testicle "arrested" along its normal pathway of descent. Maldescended = ectopic = a normal testicle abnormally placed. Cryptorchid implies hidden testicle, impalpable, generally abnormal, and found in the inguinal canal or abdomen.
Retractile testicle = normal testicle with a normally developed scrotum which retracts on minimal stimulus; it can be coaxed to lie at the base of the scrotum without undue tension.

351 An indirect hernia where the posterior wall of the sac is extra-peritoneal. Thus on the right typically the caecum herniates down, and on the left the sigmoid colon.

352 Those who have had the disease for more than ten years - especially those who have had an ileo-rectal anastomosis. Those who presented with the disease at an early age. Those with extensive colitis.

353 Nephrolithotomy nowadays should generally mean multiple calicotomies performed in conjunction with a pyelolithotomy via a Gil Vernay approach. They are done:
a) When a calculus can be palpated through a very thin area of cortex.
b) When there is a branched calculus, and the state of the other kidney precludes nephrectomy.
c) When a calculus lies within an inaccessible pelvis either because this is intrarenal or because access is is limited by adhesions due to a previous operation.

354 10-20 mg Vit. K_1.

355 When should early surgery be considered in a dissecting aneurysm of the aorta?

356 You are told that a patient had a fall onto the outstretched hand and shown an X-ray of the wrist taken in the A-P view. You immediately spot the fractured scaphoid, but before you comment on the X-ray what should you ask for and look for?

357 What are the basic pathological processes in the lung found in the two phases of 'Shock Lung' or Adult Respiratory Distress Syndrome?

358 What is Troisier's sign?

359 What are the physical signs of a slipped upper femoral epiphysis?

360 To which bone does renal cell carcinoma most commonly metastasize?

361 Within the sling of which muscle is it important to place the reconstructed rectum in a case of 'imperforate anus' with a high lying rectum and why?

362 What are the dangers of prolonged administration of steroids to patients with ulcerative colitis? (e.g. 20 mg Prednisolone/day for more than 6 weeks.)

355 The mainstay of treatment is anti-hypertensive treatment, and operation should be considered only when the dissection is progressive and causing either cerebral, renal or limb ischaemia.

356 This is a common pitfall for Casualty Officers. You should look for a lunate or perilunate dislocation which is best seen on the lateral view so remember to ask for it. A comparable view of the other side may be helpful.

357 a) Interstitial oedema with diffuse alveolar collapse, hypoxia, hypoxaemia, and A-V shunting.
b) Bronchopneumonia.

358 The involvement of left supraclavicular lymph nodes by metastatic tumour. (These are also called Virchow's nodes). The tumour is frequently carcinoma of bronchus or stomach.

359 Look: Normal or slight lateral rotation with slight shortening; wasting may be present but difficult to detect.

Feel: Shortening above the greater trochanter.

Move: Limitation of abduction and medial rotation. Slight pain sometimes. Positive Trendelenburg sign possible.

X-ray: Positive Trethowan's sign and Capener's sign. (N.B. always obtain a lateral view which is much easier to see the defect in.)

360 The humerus.

361 Within the pubo-rectalis sling of the levator group. To achieve rectal continence.

362 From the surgical viewpoint:- The colonic wall becomes friable, and often adherent to small gut serosa, making surgery difficult and hazardous. Infection, haemorrhage and perforation commoner.

363 An infant of 6 months presents with failure to thrive, intermittent attacks of abdominal distension with diarrhoea alternating with constipation. The infant did not pass meconium until 48 hours post delivery. What is the probable diagnosis and how would you investigate the child?

364 How would you manage such a child?

365 What causes of a raised calcium level must be excluded before entertaining the likelihood of primary hyperparathyroidism?

366 What are the current methods of treating keloids?

367 What is notable about the appearance of the bowel wall affected by diverticular disease?

368 Is vesicoureteric reflux common in prostatic obstruction?

369 What should be done for a fractured hyoid bone (probably due to attempted strangulation)?

363 Hirschsprung's disease. Barium enema. This should show the level of the aganglionic segment and is often diagnostic. The diagnosis should be confirmed by rectal biopsy, preferably using the suction biopsy method.

364 A colostomy in the ganglionic bowel confirmed by frozen section should be performed. When the bowel is deflated and healthy (between 2-3 months) a pull through procedure excising the aganglionic bowel is performed with the covering colostomy. The latter is closed when adequate anastomotic healing has taken place.

365 Sarcoidosis
Myeloma
Vitamin D overdose
Thyrotoxicosis
Milk-alkali syndrome
Other malignant disease

366 In the early stages when the keloid is developing the optimal and non-operative method is continuous pressure with a specially tailored 'Jobst' bandage for 23½ hours a day for up to six months but this is limited to areas where such a bandage doesn't interfere with function.

Alternatively, injection into the keloid of steroids may help at the risk of scar stretching and depigmentation.

For the established keloid excision and primary closure is almost certain to fail; tangential excision and grafting may succeed; radiotherapy often works but may be condemned as being hazardous for a benign condition. Excision and primary closure with instillation and repeated injection of steroids into the wound may succeed.

367 It is thickened and shortened.

368 Not usually; the bladder muscle hypertrophies and tends to improve the function of the vesicoureteric junction's flap-valve mechanism.

369 A tracheostomy because the incidence of glottic oedema is high.

370 Do pseudocysts of the pancreas often regress spontaneously?

371 What are the complications of a pancreatic pseudocyst?

372 What are the two common causes of pigmentation of the lining of the large and small bowel?

373 In the elderly, what is the common aetiology of a fractured neck of femur?

374 What does "primum non nocere" mean?

375 What are the indications for tonsillectomy?

376 How soon should strapping and stretching of a talipes foot begin after birth?

377 What benign tumour of the stomach may ulcerate through the mucosa giving the appearance of malignancy?

370 Not often.

371 Infection
Haemorrhage (this leads to a high mortality)
Rupture
Obstruction to adjacent organs
Pancreatic ascites

372 Melanosis Coli: Melanin is found in the monocuclear cells of the lamina propria. It is associated with the use of laxatives containing anthracene such as cascara. The pigmentation disappears on stopping the laxative.

Lipofuscinosis: Lipofuscin is deposited in small bowel muscle. It is usually found in patients with diarrhoea often due to some form of malabsorption such as coeliac disease or chronic pancreatitis. It is also seen in some patients with hypoproteinaemia usually of the protein-losing-enteropathy type.

373 Bone 'fatigue'. This allows a normal stress to cause a fracture. The patient often stumbles because the neck fractures rather than fractures because he/she stumbles.

374 Above all do no harm. (Latin)

375 a) History of recurrent attacks of acute or chronic tonsillitis, often necessitating absence from school or work.
b) History of one attack of peritonsillar abscess (quinsy).
c) Str. pyogenes or Diphtheria carrier.
d) Excision biopsy for suspected malignancy.
e) Obstruction of upper airway (particularly postural apnoea duc to enlarged tonsils and adenoids in children).

376 Immediately: certainly within days - not at the next convenient out patient clinic.

377 Leiomyoma. The mucosa can become so stretched that it ulcerates centrally from ischaemia.

378 What does grade 3 muscle strength mean?

379 Which patients with carcinoma of the prostate should not usually receive stilboestrol or similar therapy?

380 You are shown a pot of the testis with a tumour in it. Which type of tumour does this description best fit?:- 'The tumour is rounded and has destroyed the whole testis, it has a white homogeneous potato-like appearance on its cut surface.'

381 A successful outcome of adrenal surgery in patients with hypertension, aldosterone excess and low plasma renin concentration can be correlated with what pre-operative investigation?

382 Which is the only antimicrobial drug that achieves selective anaerobic chemotherapy?

383 Which plexus is affected by Hirschsprung's disease?

384 A sub-phrenic abscess is generally found in one of seven positions. What are these positions in surgico-anatomical terms?

385 What does the external laryngeal nerve supply?

378 It is just sufficient to overcome gravity.

379 Patients with disease confined to the primary site and producing few symptoms.
Those with serious cardiovascular disease.
Those who have already developed one or more of the serious complications of stilboestrol therapy.
(Local surgery, castration and/or radiotherapy may be used.)

380 It probably describes a seminoma. The teratoma often has cystic spaces, and may have other tissues such as cartilage within it. (The differential diagnosis is granulomatous orchitis.)

381 A pre-operative hypotensive response to spirolactone.

382 Metronidazole (Flagyl). N.B. Clindamycin and lincomycin are also active against most staph. aureus and most streptococci, but not against strep. faecalis. The only other commonly used antimicrobials active against some anaerobes are penicillin, tetracycline, erythromycin, rifamicin and chloramphenicol.

383 Both 'Auter' (Auerbach's) and Middle (Meissner's) lack ganglion cells.

384 Right
Supra-hepatic Anterior
Posterior
Infra-hepatic Anterior
Posterior
(hepato-renal pouch)

Left
Supra-hepatic
Antero-hepatic
Lesser sac.

385 Inferior constrictor and cricothyroid muscles.

386 How would you classify the fractures sustained by a fall on the outstretched hand?

387 What is the differential diagnosis of a sacrococcygeal tumour?

388 When performing radical excision of a malignant melanoma from the calf of a patient and covering the defect with a split-thickness skin graft, from where do you obtain the skin usually?

389 List the causes of a localised hepatic swelling?

390 Pre-operative assessment of lung function is important before any major thoracic or lung operation. Which tests would you find useful?

391 Name three drugs used to treat hypotonic bladder.

392 Whose operation may slightly improve the prognosis of a patient with polycystic kidneys?

393 Is the plasma gastrin level elevated in either G.U. or D.U. patients?

386 Classify them according to age:-

0 - 12 yr.	greenstick fracture of the radius and ulna
12 - 16 yr.	fractured distal radial epiphysis ('juvenile Colles')
16 - 35 yr.	fractured scaphoid
35 - 55 yr.	fractured shaft of humerus
55 yrs. +	Colles fracture

387 A low meningocele
Chordoma
Neuroblastoma
Hamartoma (Lipoma or angioma)
Cystic duplication of the rectum
Postrectal abscess

388 The thigh of the opposite leg.

389 Secondary tumour
Reidel's lobe
Hydatid cyst
Amoebic abscess
Hepatoma

390 Ask the patient to walk up a flight of steps and see how breathless he becomes.
Measure vital capacity (V.C.).
Estimate Peak Expiratory Flow Rate (P.E.F.R.).
Forced Expiratory Volume in 1 sec. (F.E.V.$_1$).
Blood gases of which P_{CO_2} is the most important (i.e. under 45)

391 Carbachol, 'Mestinon' - pyridostigmine bromide, 'Ubretid'- distigmine bromide.

392 Rovsing's deroofing of the cysts.

393 Yes. In G.U. patients but seldom D.U. patients.

394 What % of patients with hyperparathyroidism have M.E.A. Type 1?

395 What is the best age to examine for cryptorchidism?

396 Give four causes of mesenteric cysts.

397 Where are the crypts of Luschka found?

398 What is cholesterosis?

399 What are the possible alternative methods of treating a patient with Dupuytren's contracture?

400 What are the X-ray markings of the ileal mesentery?

401 What muscles are excised in a block dissection of the neck?

402 What are the common causes of chronic epididymo-orchitis?

394 About 15 - 20%. The measurement of mean fasting gastrin level may distinguish those with a gastrinoma because it will be much higher than normal.

395 The first year of life when the cremasteric muscle can always be overcome to diagnose a retractile testis.

396 Chylo-lymphatic, commonest and often in the ileal mesentery.
Enterogenous, sequestration of gut or reduplication - it may have a ciliated lining and thick wall.
Urogenital remnant.
Dermoid or omental cyst

397 In the gall bladder.

398 An asymptomatic mucosal hyperplasia of the gall bladder often compared to a strawberry appearance, due to deposition of cholesterol crystals in histiocytes in the mucosa.

399 a) Do nothing, i.e. treat nodules alone only if they cause disabling pain or interfere with function. There is little or no evidence to recommend 'prophylactic surgery'.
b) Percutaneous fasciotomy.
c) Limited palmar fasciectomy.
d) Open palmar fasciectomy or fasciectomy with skin closure direct or with skin graft or skin flap.
e) Fasciectomy without attempt to close the defect - open palm technique.
f) Amputation of the affected digit with or without amputation through the metacarpal 'ray amputation'.

400 Transverse process of L.2 to the right sacro iliac joint.

401 Sternomastoid and omo-hyoid (and lateral strap muscles if indicated).

402 Tuberculosis affecting the globus minor is the classical cause, but half treated or indolent descending infection can produce a similar picture.

403 What criteria are used to judge that an intestinal obstruction is resolving during conservative treatment?

404 What is the differential diagnosis in cases of an asymptomatic patient in whom a well circumscribed pulmonary opacity (Coin lesion) is discovered on routine X-ray examination?

405 What is Kehr's sign?

406 What is this a classical description of?- 'A wasted, puny, pot-bellied child, chronically constipated with visible peristalsis, distended abdomen with audible tympanitic sounds, who suffers from bouts of vomiting, but seldom soils his nappies'.

407 What is the difference between primary and secondary bile salts?

408 Which age group, and which side do varicoceles usually affect?

409 Which of the paraduodenal fossae is the commonest one associated with a small bowel obstruction?

410 What do you understand by the term 'occult carcinoma of the breast'?

403 Lessening gastric aspiration.
Normal bowel sounds.
Passage of flatus or bowel actions.
Loss of pain if present previously.
Fall in pulse rate.
X-ray evidence of decreased distension, loss of gas-fluid levels and onward transmission of bowel contents.

404 Bronchial carcinoma
Single pulmonary metastatic deposit
Bronchial adenoma
Hamartoma
Cyst
T.B. focus

405 Hyperaesthesia at the left shoulder tip associated with splenic rupture. (O'Connell's modification is to produce this hyperaesthesia by elevating the foot of the bed.)

406 A child with Hirschsprung's disease.

407 Primary are synthesized, conjugated with glycine or taurine, and secreted in the bile by an active transport mechanism.

Secondary are produced from primary bile salts by the action of intestinal bacteria; some are absorbed and participate in the enterohepatic circulation. Some are insoluble and are excreted in the faeces.

408 Teenagers or young adults, on the left side.

409 The left duodeno-jejunal fossa (carries the inferior mesenteric vein in its free margin).

410 Carcinoma of the breast in which metastases are evident clinically before the primary tumour is detected.

411 Outline your answer to the question "Discuss the treatment of an elderly patient with a hip fracture".

412 Why is a tarso-metatarsal dislocation potentially a very serious injury?

413 Is is possible to distinguish clinically between a myelocoele and a meningo-myelocoele?

414 In a case of Wilm's tumour, how long a recurrence free period suggests a cure?

415 Patients are often referred to the Out Patient Clinic as having suffered a 'painful attack of bleeding piles.' What do you think of this as a diagnosis?

416 What is the optimal site for percutaneous splenic puncture?

417 What % of patients with myasthenia gravis have a thymic tumour?

411 "Discuss the treatment" assumes that the patient is already in hospital, history taken, examined and investigated. You should discuss the indications and contra-indications for conservative/operative care including the types of operation. Finally discuss postoperative management, complications and their treatment.

Conservative management
(i) Patient unfit for anaesthetic
(ii) Inadequate facilities for operation

Fracture Types
Intracapsular a) subcapital b) transcervical
Extracapsular a) basal cervical b) trochanteric

Treatments
Intracapsular: (i) prosthetic replacement in the elderly with displaced fractures
(ii) reduction and pinning in the younger ones or those with no displacement

Extracapsular: pin and plate

Postop. Care Early mobilisation, physiotherapy, anti DVT
Complications Haemorrhage, infection, DVT/PE, fat embolism, pressure sores, urinary retention
Rehabilitation

412 It can endanger the blood supply to the foot and thus requires emergency reduction.

413 There is no reliable clinical differentiation between them.

414 Two years *(Platt and Linden 1964 Cancer 17 1573.)*

415 The vast majority of haemorrhoids bleed painlessly or with only minor discomfort. Severe pain associated with bleeding is much more typical of anal fissure or rarely thrombosed piles or carcinoma.

416 Intercostal space, midaxillary line, in inspiration.

417 About 14-16%. *(Keynes 1955 B.J.S. 42 449)*

418 Why should all inguinal herniae in infants be managed surgically?

419 What conditions predispose to Shock Lung?

420 The congenital defects at the umbilicus termed 'exomphalos' may be subdivided into three groups. What are these?

421 Describe the action of Cimetidine on the stomach.

422 What is the basic argument for using radiotherapy rather than surgery in the first instance in the treatment of advanced carcinoma of the larynx?

423 Which renal lesions may simulate a nephroblastoma clinically?

424 What sort of history may precede a sigmoid volvulus?

418 There is a very high risk of incarceration, resulting in strangulation of the intestine in the male or of the ovary and Fallopian tube in the female. Testicular atrophy may be a late sequel of incarceration.
(Atwell, J. D. Paediatric Surgery in Operative Surgery, Rob & Smith, 3rd Edition. Butterworths. Page 1)

419 Sepsis: Peritonitis, soft tissue infection, pulmonary infection, pancreatitis, burn sepsis.

Shock/Trauma: needing massive fluid or blood replacement
thoracic or cerebral trauma
fat embolism

Miscellaneous: Cardio-pulmonary by-pass
aspiration
O_2 toxicity
renal transplantation

420 Hernia into the cord (persistence of physiological hernia)
Omphalocoele (failure of mesoderm to complete formation of anterior abdominal wall)
Gastroschisis (probably an early rupture of the sac of a physiological hernia)

421 It is a Histamine H_2 Receptor Antagonist and inhibits resting and stimulated gastric acid secretion.

422 In terms of survival X.R.T. provides 40% cure by itself as measured at five years, whereas surgery gives a 70% five year survival but patient loses his voice. However, of the X.R.T. failures 70% will have a five year survival if given surgery also (i.e. total laryngectomy).

423 Neuroblastoma
Hydronephrosis
Cystic kidneys
Solitary renal cysts
Renal vein thrombosis
Pyonephrosis

424 Usually a long history of attacks of abdominal pain with constipation followed by diarrhoea and copious flatus with the relief of pain.

425 Define a hamartoma.

426 What are the basic steps of a Keller's operation?

427 What is the Pierre-Robin syndrome, and what is the main problem in initial management?

428 Describe a juvenile rectal polyp.

429 Under what circumstances would you choose to employ bi-polar coagulation in preference to ordinary coagulation diathermy?

430 Which type of gastric carcinoma has a 75% five year survival?

431 What are the two main types of forceps used for reducing a displaced nasal fracture?

432 What is the commonest congenital malformation?

433 What type of infant elective tracheostomy tube is required to ensure normal development of the larynx?

425 A hamartoma is a non-neoplastic malformation characterised by an abnormal mixture or overgrowth of tissues indigenous to the part with an excess of one or more of these.

426 Keller's operation is for bunion. Most surgeons employ tourniquet (exsanguination of the limb). Excise the proximal third of the proximal phalanx of the great toe to make a pseudarthrosis and chisel off the exostosis of the first metatarsal head. The foot may be bandaged immobile, plastered or left free according to choice.

427 Cleft palate, associated with mandibular retrognathia, leading to severe feeding and respiratory problems. Tongue swallowing demands special nursing.

428 A bright red, smooth, glistening sphere, which contains large cystic areas filled with mucin. The rest is mainly connective tissue with fewer epithelial tubules than in an adenomatous polyp.

429 When attempting to achieve haemostasis in an organ or part effectively served by an end-artery; i.e. a digit, the penis, the eye etc. Bi-polar coagulation is safer in these circumstances as the current passes by the shortest route between the blades of the bi-polar coagulation forceps which grip the bleeding point, whereas the current has to pass along the length of the extremity when using ordinary diathermy.

430 A purely mucosal carcinoma. (It may be widespread but it fails to invade through the muscularis mucosae.) Recent work in Japan has drawn attention to this potentially curable condition.

431 Walsham's and Ashes'

432 Talipes. (2.8/1000 total births.)

433 One with a fenestration in the shoulder and an expiratory valve (e.g. Alder Hey tube) to ensure that the expiratory tide passes through the larynx.

434 Which solid tumours can be nowadays treated with chemotherapy with a reasonable hope of cure?

435 What is the treatment of a neonatal duodenal obstruction?

436 What are the typical findings on lymphography in primary lymphoedema?

437 What factors predispose to dislocation of the patella?

438 What are the essential points about a bimanual examination of the bladder for suspected tumour?

439 What does this description refer to?
'Naked eye appearance'. There are two chief types, the hard sclerosing type is usually comparatively localised and by its growth round the ...., and the resulting contraction, a considerable degree of stenosis is produced. The soft or encephaloid type involves a greater extent of the ...., forms irregular projections into the lumen, and thus tends to cause occlusion. The tumour frequently spreads in the submucous tissue, and forms secondary growths which raise up the mucosa, giving an appearance of multifocal origin.

440 What are the microscopic appearances of such a tumour?

441 In which part of the bronchial tree does a small inhaled foreign body usually lodge?

434 Burkitt's Lymphoma
Choriocarcinoma
Disseminated Hodgkins
Mycosis Fungoides

435 Duodenoduodenostomy or duodenojejunostomy.

436 Diffuse hypoplasia of the lymphatics although varicose lymphatics, dermal backflow, and even chylous reflux may be present.

437 Small high patella
Female sex
Usually low lateral femoral condyles
Ligamentous laxity
Knock-knees
Internal rotation of the legs

438 The patient's muscles must be completely relaxed under general anaesthesia. Remember to feel high up for lesions of the fundus and close behind the pubic symphysis for anterior tumours.
Repeat the bimanual examination after resection of the tumour and record the clinical stage.

439 Carcinoma of the oesophagus.

440 In most cases the tumour is a poorly keratinised squamous carcinoma; rarely it resembles oat-celled bronchial carcinoma. Adenocarcinoma also has been described, but many of these are due to extension of a gastric carcinoma.

441 Right posterior basal bronchus.

442 What are the recommended tests for confirming brain death assuming that?

1) The patient is deeply comatose and there is no suspicion that this is due to depressant drugs, hypothermia, metabolic or endocrine disturbance.
2) The patient is on a respirator because spontaneous respiration has become inadequate or has ceased.
3) That there is no doubt that the patient's condition is due to irreversible structural brain damage and that a diagnosis of a disorder which can lead to brain death should have been established.

443 With which renal disease is vesico-ureteric reflux most commonly associated?

444 Which members of the African races are particularly prone to skin cancers?

445 What operative procedure may be carried out for an obstructing lesion of the ascending colon?

446 Williams recently emphasised the importance of swelling of what part of the brain as a cause of failure to improve in cases of closed head injury? (*B.J.S. 1976 63 169-172).*

447 What are the possible symptoms and signs of hypocalcaemia?

442 Basically the absence of brain stem reflexes must be shown. This entails:-

a) Fixed pupils, unreactive to light.
b) Absent corneal reflex.
c) Absent vestibulo-ocular reflex (20 ml of ice-cold water squirted into the patent ext. aud. meatus).
d) No somatic reflexes.
e) No gag reflex.
f) No respiratory movement on disconnection of the respirator provided the P_{CO_2} is greater than 50 mmHg.

(check by blood gases, or give mixture of 5% CO_2+ O_2 via ventilator for five minutes following 10 minutes of pure O_2, and then give O_2 at 6 L/min via intra-tracheal catheter).

N.B. Make sure that the patient has body temperature of 35°C or more, and if in doubt repeat the test 24 hours later. E.E.G. and cerebral angiography are not necessary.

443 Chronic pyelonephritis. There is some dispute over which is cause and effect: reflux + infection in children = pyelonephritis + scarring; sterile reflux may be harmless, although many surgeons would operate to correct gross reflux.

444 Albinos. Many die in adolescence and early adulthood from squamous cell carcinomata.

445 Immediate right hemicolectomy with primary ileo-transverse anastomosis, or for an inexperienced surgeon, a side to side ileo-transverse by-pass anastomosis with caecostomy to avoid a difficult hemicolectomy.

446 Temporal lobe swelling. N.B. If the temporal lobe is massively swollen and damaged, adequate decompression may involve resection of the temporal lobe.

447 The renal concentrating ability is depressed which leads to polyuria and polydipsia; lethargy, constipation vomiting hypotonia, bone pain, muscle cramps, abdominal pain, muscle weakness, psychosis. (Remember;'Stones, bones and abdominal groans'.

448 List some of the causes of recurrent laryngeal nerve paralysis.

449 What is the treatment for a primary ureteric carcinoma?

450 What advice should you give the parent of a child who is found to develop a strawberry naevus on a cheek at the age of two weeks?

451 Why are clinical manifestations of renal tuberculosis rare in childhood?

452 What is the likely cause of a recurrent preauricular abscess?

453 What is the effect of damage to the external laryngeal nerve?

448 Unknown aetiology 30%.
Central lesions, i.e. tabes, diseases affecting the medulla.
Peripheral: traumatic, including surgical damage (thyroidectomy/patent ductus op.).

Inflammatory - a - polyneuritis, beri-beri
b - infective - diphtheria
typhoid
streptococcal
virus - herpetic
c - toxic - lead

Neoplasia - carcinoma of bronchus
carcinoma of the larynx and thyroid
carcinoma of upper oesophagus
carcinoma or other malignant disease of mediastinal lymph nodes

Degenerative - aneurysm of aortic arch.

449 Controversial. Provided the patient has a normal functioning contralateral renal tract, the standard treatment is nephroureterectomy taking a cuff of bladder with followup of the rest of the urothelium. If the tumour were localised and not invasive, some would attempt excision with anastomosis and renal conservation.

450 That unless it interferes with vision of the adjacent eye it should be left alone. These naevi often enlarge rapidly for a few months, then stabilise and then gradually regress after about one to two years. The sign of regression is the grey-purple sclerosis of the surface epithelium and diminution in size. The final appearance is often of only a small blemish. Occasionally excision of redundant lax skin folds in the site of the regressed naevus may be indicated.

451 Unlike most of the other extra-pulmonary manifestations of tuberculosis, the clinical symptoms and signs of renal infection usually take between five and fifteen years to appear after primary infection.

452 Presence of an epithelial track - preauricular sinus.

453 Usually only slight alteration in laryngeal tone which may be transient.

454 Chronic atherosclerotic mesenteric vascular insufficiency is often the cause of pain after meals and what else?

455 In rheumatoid disease inability to extend the wrist joint actively may be caused by which two types of pathology?

456 With which type of injury is posterior urethral damage usually associated?

457 What does neurolysis mean?

458 Is C.D.H. more or less common in premature babies?

459 List some of the X-ray signs of a right sub-phrenic abscess.

460 How important is the size of the perineal haematoma in a case of ruptured urethra?

461 When gastro-colic fistula occurs it is generally a complication of which conditions?

462 Is active disease a contraindication for surgery of the rheumatoid hand?

463 What should be arranged for a patient en route for the operating theatre prior to a pyelo- or ureterolithotomy?

454 Malabsorption, weight loss, and these symptoms may be the prelude to massive bowel infarction.

455 Extensor tendon rupture.
Entrapment neuropathy of the posterior interosseous nerve.

456 Central fracture of the pelvic ring or any pelvic fracture with dislocation.

457 Freeing of a nerve from surrounding structures, e.g. scar tissue.

458 Less common. (Probably because of lower exposure to maternal ligament relaxing hormone.)

459 Raised right hemi-diaphragm.
Immobile hemi-diaphragm on inspir-expiration films or screening.
Fluid level (gas within) an abscess.
Pleural effusion ± other chest signs.
Fixity of the renal outline on standing, due to inflammation, seen best on I.V.U.

460 Unimportant: The whole envelope of the bulb of the corpus spongiosum may be ruptured with an intact urethral epithelium.

461 Most commonly: Carcinoma or reticulosis
Crohn's disease
Gastric surgery especially recurrent ulceration after gastro-enterostomy.

462 No. However most surgeons prefer to carry out reconstructive or salvage surgery in the absence of active disease. There is little evidence that surgery actually causes a flare-up of the disease.

463 A plain X-ray of the abdomen to check that the stone has not moved significantly since the previous X-ray examination.

464 Discuss the importance of incompetent valves in aetiology of varicose veins.

465 What observations should be made in the notes after performing a sigmoidoscopy examination?

466 What is the best operative management of traumatic colonic injury?
Ref: Shennan J. 1973 B.J.S. 60 673. Seat belt injuries of the left colon.
Freeark R.J. 1977 J. Trauma 17 563.

467 In a radical cancer operation for carcinoma of the stomach, what should be removed?

468 You operate on a 35 year old woman for appendicitis and you find not only acute appendicitis but also a 5 cm diameter solid round mass in the left ovary. What should you do?

469 Are most urinary stones radio-opaque and biliary ones lucent, or is it the other way round? Does the answer have any implications for patient management?

470 Injury to the cricoid cartilage in performing a tracheostomy may lead to what problem?

471 How is carcinoma of the transverse colon treated?

464 Two types of incompetence are described. Primary due to physical damage to the valves, and secondary due to excessive flow leading to dilatation of the vein and thus failure of approximation of valve cusps. One of the basic premises of injection sclerotherapy is that obliteration of the primarily incompetent valves will lead to regression of the secondary incompetence of other undamaged valves.

465 Luminal contents.
Size of lumen,any narrowing or ballooning.
Mucosal appearances including contact bleeding, polyps.
Height achieved, any difficulty encountered.
Response of the patient.
Any blood: free intraluminal or mixed with faeces.
Gross incontinence of the air introduced during the examination.

466 Exteriorisation of the affected bowel with or without resection is the safest method. Primary resection and anastomosis with proximal decompression leads to an unacceptably high sepsis rate.

467 En-bloc removal of 80-90% or even 100% of the stomach, the spleen, distal half of pancreas, both omenta, and the pancreatic subpyloric hepatic and coeliac lymph nodes.

468 At this age, a 5 cm solid tumour in an ovary should be a benign teratoma (dermoid cyst) or a fibroma. The ovary should be removed, if the tumour is malignant, a gynaecologist should be consulted.

469 Most urinary stones are radio-opaque and biliary ones lucent. In consequence, patients with renal calculi can be followed by serial plain X-rays, whereas those with gall stones require repeated contrast radiographs.

470 Sub-glottic stenosis.

471 Either: immediate resection with primary anastomosis
or excision of the tumour and mesentery with a spur colostomy
or caecostomy, proximal colostomy or ileostomy with later resection.

472 What does a urate stone look and feel like?

473 What does the string sign of Kantor refer to?

474 Describe the operation of excision of a pharyngeal pouch.

475 What are the main complications of an anal pull-through operation?

476 Meconium ileus may be treated by gastrograffin enema: What other lesion of the infant bowel may also be treated by an enema of radiographic contrast medium?

477 Which type of fractured neck of femur is commonly missed?

478 What is the commonest type of oesophageal atresia?

479 What is the sex incidence of laryngeal carcinoma?

472 Yellow crystalline and hard.

473 The narrowing of the terminal ileal lumen in Crohn's disease as seen on barium meal follow-through.

474 To identify the oesophageal opening the patient is asked to swallow a small weight on a thread 24 hours prior to surgery. Under a general anaesthetic, the patient is placed supine on the table with neck extended. The patient is endoscoped and the pouch identified and packed with ½" ribbon gauze soaked in proflavine. Through an oblique incision along the anterior border of the left sterno-mastoid, (or transverse incision at the level of the cricoid) the lateral lobe of the thyroid is mobilised, necessitating ligation of the middle thyroid veins and if necessary the inferior thyroid artery. The thyroid is retracted forward and carotid sheath backward. The sac packed with gauze can be easily identified. It is freed from surrounding tissues, and a small incision made into the fundus of the sac to allow separation of the wall of the sac from the mucous membrane. The pouch is resected at its neck and a cricopharyngeal myotomy is carried out. The oesophagus is repaired in two layers, aided by the previous splitting of the wall into its two components. An N/G tube is then passed. The neck is closed with suction drainage. Post operatively the patient is fed by N/G tube which is usually removed after 7-10 days.

475 Necrosis of the colon followed by haemorrhage.
Pelvic abscess.
Stenosis of colo-anal junction.
Incontinence - from stretch injury to the internal (and possibly external) sphincter.

476 Intussusception by barium enema.

477 An impacted fracture.

478 80% have a blind upper pouch and a fistula between the trachea and distal pouch.

479 10 males to 1 female.

480 What interpretation would you put on the following results of gastric function in a patient?
Low basal acid output
Low insulin induced acid output
High acid output following Pentagastrin stimulation

481 Approximately 80% of bladder tumours arise in which part of the bladder?

482 A middle aged woman complaining of frequency, nocturia, and severe suprapubic pain, with her urine free of pus cells, and bacteriologically sterile, who on cystoscopy has a contracted bladder is probably suffering from what? What may be seen on cystoscopy?

483 What incision is usually made for a tracheo-oesophageal fistula repair?

484 After entering the thorax what is the first important structure to be divided in such an operation?

485 What medical advice might be given to a patient with polycystic kidneys?

486 Where is the site of constriction in a strangulated indirect inguinal hernia?

487 Distinguish the embryological origins of branchial cyst and fistula.

488 Which laboratory tests are used to establish a diagnosis of D.I.C.? (disseminated intravascular coagulation.)

489 What is a probable cause of dyspnoea and cyanosis following tracheostomy if the airway is apparently clear?

480 The patient has a large parietal cell mass, but no obvious vagal or gastrin drive e.g. complete vagotomy.

481 The base, adjacent to the ureteric orifices.

482 Chronic interstitial cystitis. She may also notice haematuria intermittently. On cystoscopy a 'Hunner's Ulcer' may be seen in the vault. Splitting of the mucosa on hydrodistension is typical.

483 Right postero-lateral approach through 5th rib space or bed of the latter with the baby prone, or semi prone.

484 The azygos vein.

485 Drink a lot of water.
Low protein diet.
Take iron for anaemia (of dubious efficacy).
Check urine frequently for infection.

486 It can be at the internal or external ring, or at the neck of the sac, or may be due to bands within the sac.

487 Cyst: Is derived from the endoderm of the second branchial pouch.

Fistula: Is derived from a pre-cervical sinus, which is an epithelially lined space of the second and third clefts.

488 Fibrin degradation products, FDP: increased.
Fibrinogen level: decreased.
Thrombin clotting time, TT: increased.
Platelets: reduced.

489 Mediastinal emphysema, associated with tight skin stitches around the tube.

490 What are the causes of blood stained fluid (not free blood) in the peritoneal cavity in a patient with NO history of trauma?

491 What is the usual formula for calculating the alkali requirements of a patient knowing the base excess?

492 Describe the operation of closure of colostomy.

493 The sabre tibia of syphilis is due to which pathological process? Compare Rickets and Paget's disease.

494 What is the arterial supply of the femoral head?

490 Acute pancreatitis
Mesenteric embolus
Acute intestinal obstruction (often with strangulation)
Torsion of a viscus
Ruptured aneurysm (early or partial tear)
Primary streptococcal peritonitis

491 1/3 body weight in Kg X Base Excess = Total alkali needs in MEq.
N.B. Give 1/2 requirement initially and then the body may begin to compensate for itself.

492 The need of bowel preparation is arguable, with variation from full preparation to none at all. General anaesthesia. Skin prep. Supine patient. Skin drapes. Incision: around the edge of the colostomy taking a small rim of skin with the bowel. Stay sutures are inserted through the mucucutaneous junction to aid control of colon with slight traction. The incision is deepened all round through subcutaneous fat and muscles. The general peritoneal cavity is opened early and the colon dissected distally and proximally for several centimetres so that the colostomy is now fully mobile. The skin edge is now trimmed as much as possible to freshen the edges of the anastomosis allowing the edges to unroll. It doesn't matter if small portions of skin are sewn in. If the distal lumen seems too narrow, then enlarge it by a longitudinal cut. Some surgeons perform a formal resection of the colostomy with end to end anastomosis, but this is frequently very bloody and probably unnecessary. Closure may be one or two layer, continuous or interrupted. Surgeons hold strongly differing views about these details. Most use unabsorbable sutures in at least one layer. It is advisable to drain the abdomen,and close with a few loose sutures.

493 Diffuse tertiary syphilis causes periostitis, with laying down of new bone causing pseudo-bowing. Paget's and rickets cause truly bent bones.

494 a) Reflected vessels from the capsule - often torn in a displaced fracture leading to avascular necrosis of the head.
b) Medullary cavity vessels from the shaft.
c) Small and variable amount through the ligamentum teres.

495 What degree of negative nitrogen balance occurs immediately following an operation such as vagotomy and pyloroplasty?

496 List some of the important points about the technique of large bowel anastomosis.

497 What is the commonest site for a pulsion diverticulum of the bladder?

498 What is the first of a two stage urethral reconstruction in a case of subcoronal hypospadias?

499 What is the incidence of leakage following colostomy closure?

500 The diagnosis of pyloric stenosis is often delayed or missed in premature infants. Why?

501 What nevertheless clinches the diagnosis?

502 What are the recognised causes of pneumaturia?

495 About 10 g/day. (In severe burn it might be as much as 20-25 g nitrogen per day)

496 There should be no tension either on the bowel or on the sutures.
There should be a visibly good blood supply to both cut edges of bowel.
Always drain the abdomen.
If in doubt about the anastomosis create a temporary proximal colostomy.
The method of suture is controversial. In general do what is safest in your hands - if a two layer closure is used, one layer should probably be of non-absorbable suture material.

497 Just supero-lateral to one of the ureteric orifices. It can lead to obstruction of the ureter in this position.

498 The chordee (ventral curvature of the penile shaft) must be eliminated by thorough excision of its tight fascial or fibrous bands. Closure of the defect so created may be by Z-plasty, local flaps of foreskin, or simply skin closure in a direction 90° to the original incision, this may also necessitate a dorsal tension releasing incision. The release of the chordee will cause the urinary meatus to come to lie closer to the base of the penile shaft.

499 This is a controversial subject. *Knox, Birkett and Collins, Closure of Colostomy, B.J.S. (1971) 58 669-672* suggested 25% incidence of leakage. This received a critical press. The St. Mark's figures are of around a 2% incidence - but this reflects selected patients in a specialised unit.

500 The premature infant is often anorexic rather than hungry and vomiting is often regurgitant rather than projectile. Visible peristalsis is not an abnormal feature of the premature.

501 A palpable lump. (Best felt during or immediately after a feed.

502 Most cases are due to vesico-colic fistula; pneumaturia can occur as a rare complication of urinary infection in diabetes due to glucose fermentation by gas forming organisms.

503 The principles of treatment of shock lung are to treat the underlying cause of the condition, give O_2 therapy assisted ventilation with or without intubation or tracheostomy. What important maneouvre may you have to institute with the respirator?

504 Which haemorrhoids are regarded as unsuitable for injection treatment?

505 What is the conservative treatment of patients with lymphoedema due to hypoplastic lymphatics?

506 What is the organism usually responsible for osteomyelitis?

507 What X-ray sign indicates skeletal maturity?

508 Define a laryngocoele.

509 Most carcinomata of the bladder are of transitional cell type. What are the other possible types that are rarer?

510 What is the classical presentation of a choledochal cyst?

503 Raise the P.E.E.P. (Post expiratory end pressure) but beware of pneumothorax.

504 Fourth and third degree haemorrhoids.
Failure of conservative treatment of 2nd degree haemorrhoids.
Piles which have already thrombosed and fibrosed.
Intero-external piles.
When arterial pulsation is palpable or visible in the pedicle.

505 Elastic stockings, worn constantly.
Elevation of the legs at night.
Intermittent diuretics.
Penicillin to prevent cellulitis.
At all times prevent chronic swelling which leads to irreversible changes.

506 Staphylococcus aureus in 90% of cases.

507 Risser's. (Fusion of the posterior superior iliac crest apophyses.)

508 A narrow necked, air containing, diverticulum resulting from the herniation of laryngeal mucosa. It originates in the laryngeal sacculus situated in the anterior 1/3 of the laryngeal ventricle and ascending between the false cord and ala of the thyroid. It may herniate through the thyro-hyoid membrane and present as a mass in the neck in which case it is known as an external laryngocoele. If it remains within the bounds of the larynx then it is an internal laryngocoele.

509 Squamous cell carcinoma (stones, bilharzia, leukoplakia).
Adenocarcinoma (urachal origin, or metaplasia).
Very rare: sarcoma bothyroides, lymphoma, secondaries.

510 Abdominal pain; vague intermittent.
Jaundice; often fluctuant in degree.
Palpable abdominal mass; also often fluctuant.

511 What does Boas' sign indicate?

512 Why does blood not clot in the pleural cavity?

513 What is a Smith's fracture?

514 What is the major complication of untreated choledochal cyst?

515 What are the particular problems associated with the treatment of a fracture of the shaft of the tibia?

516 How long is the adult ureter?

517 What is a bunion?

518 How long can a complete intestinal obstruction be treated conservatively?

519 In what way does the type of incision into the trachea in a tracheostomy procedure differ in an infant from an adult?

520 Which neurogenic tumours may arise in close proximity to the ribs?

511 Hyperaesthesia at the lower angle of the right scapula associated with cholecystitis.

512 It is defibrinated by the movement of the heart and lungs. Only in massive haemorrhage does the blood clot.

513 A reversed Colles' fracture. Look carefully to see whether it goes into the wrist joint. A Smith's fracture must be reduced in full supination and held in an above elbow P.O.P. (The reduction is totally different from that used for a Colles' fracture.

514 Biliary cirrhosis with recurrent ascending cholangitis.

515 Skin: The fracture is frequently compound and there is often skin loss making closure difficult particularly if bone is exposed. Risk of infection is high and is compounded by relatively poor blood supply in this region. Bone: There is a slow rate of healing, with high incidence of delayed or non-union. There is greater difficulty in controlling the deformity than in most other fractures.

516 Approximately 25 cm (divided equally above and below by the pelvic brim).

517 An inflamed adventitious bursa overlying an exostosis. (Generally in relation to the head of the first metatarsal.)

518 Usually not more than 24 hours, preferably within 12 hours in which time fluid and electrolyte disturbances can be largely corrected.

519 In the infant avoid removing any cartilage: a straight vertical incision will minimise the risk of subglottic stenosis. In an adult a circle of cartilage should be excised or a Björk flap cut.

520 Neurofibroma. (From the intercostal nerve.) Ganglioneuroma. (From the sympathetic chain.)

521 What single type of pathological lesion may cause?
In the elderly: visual loss, dementia, raised I.C.P.
In the young and middle-aged: visual field changes or loss, and hypopituitism.
In the adolescent: endocrine abnormalities.
In children and infants: symptoms of raised I.C.P. i.e. headaches, vomiting, sudden onset of squinting.

522 What may you see (or not see) on a plain X-ray of chest and upper abdomen which is suggestive of achalasia of the oesophagus?

523 What numerical figures are important in performing oesophagoscopy on an adult?

524 To which organ is the cytotoxic agent Daunorubicin particularly toxic?

525 Distinguish the pathology underlying an osteochondral fracture from that in osteochondritis dissecans.

526 What six symptoms and signs may be present in an intussusception?

527 What other technique, other than operation, can be used to reduce an intussusception? What are the contraindications?

528 What operations are currently popular in the treatment of Hirschsprung's disease once a protective colostomy has been created?

521 Craniopharyngioma.

522 Probably absent gastric air bubble.
Possibly air or air/fluid level in the oesophagus.

523 15 cm (Cricopharyngeus)
25 cm (Aortic arch)
40 cm (Cardia)

524 The heart.

525 An osteochondral fracture involves normal bone and is due to a single traumatic episode. In osteochondritis dissecans a fragment of articular cartilage together with subchondral bone becomes partly or completely separated from the joint surface, the plane of separation occurring through ischaemic bone.

526 Vomiting: Colicky abdominal pain: Presence of a mass per abdomen: Emptiness in the right iliac fossa: Presence of blood on rectal examination or passage of red currant jelly: Fever.

527 The barium enema technique. It should not be used if there is:-
1) peritonism/peritonitis.
2) history of longer than 24 hours.
3) presence of fluid levels on plain X-ray.
4) clinically ill child.

528 a) Duhamel's *(1960 Archs. Dis. Childhood* 35 *38)*
b) Swenson's *(1964 Ann. Surg.* 160 *540)*
c) Soave's *(1964 Archs. Dis. Childhood* 39 *116)*
d) Rehbein's *(1960 Archs. Dis. Childhood* 35 *29)*

529 In which rare circumstances can an appendix be excised without leaving an abdominal scar?

530 What are the commonly used operations for recurrent dislocation of the patella?

531 Which area of skin is supplied by the ilio-inguinal nerve (which can be accidentally cut or damaged in a herniorraphy or orchidopexy)?

532 What may cause pain and restriction of movement after hip replacement?

533 At which site does carcinoma of the colon have the worst prognosis?

534 Is the marked increase in the frequency of cholecystectomy operations in the past twenty years due to an increase in the prevalence of gall stones?

535 If a patient has an arterio-venous malformation of the forearm, what may you be expected to demonstrate by simple elevation of the arm?

536 Why was the Paul-Mickulicz procedure introduced in colonic surgery?

537 Apart from the histology which is essential to diagnosis, what clinical features often help to distinguish Crohn's disease from ulcerative colitis of the large bowel?

529 The inverted appendix may be the apex of an intussusception presenting at the rectum which is subsequently reduced hydrostatically.

530 a) Medial capsule reefing and lateral release.
b) Tibial tubercle transfer distally and medially.

It is sometime necessary to combine these procedures with patellectomy for a badly worn posterior surface; patellectomy alone as the definitive procedure is not satisfactory because the extensor expansion continues itself to dislocate.

531 The ilio-inguinal nerve supplies the skin of the anterior abdominal wall over the pubic symphysis, of the thigh over the proximal and medial part of the femoral triangle, and of the upper part of the scrotum, root and dorsum of the penis. (Labium major in the female.)

532 a) New bone formation (Men commoner than women.).
b) Loosening of either prosthesis.
c) Infection.
d) Dislocation.
e) Prosthesis fracture due to metal fatigue.

533 Splenic flexure.

534 Probably not. Studies such as Bateson's *(B.M.J. 1975 4 427-429)* suggest that the prevalence of gall stones has not changed significantly in the past 50 years.

535 That the veins fail to collapse on elevating the arm.

536 To reduce the then high mortality of end to end anastomosis of the colon.

537 Perianal disease is commoner, rectal bleeding rarer than in ulcerative colitis. On barium enema the disease is often of patchy distribution with strictures and fissures.

538 What is the histology of gynaecomastia?

539 Describe the modern treatment of talipes equinovarus.

540 Why does biliary tract cancer carry an appalling prognosis?

541 Where do sublingual dermoids present?

542 What are Eder-Puestow dilators used for?

543 What is the underlying cause of the Budd-Chiari syndrome?

544 Can thyroid tissue be aberrant in a lateral position in the neck?

545 What are the causes of a mobile kyphosis?

538 Basically no lobules but mainly ducts with fibrous tissue, some inflammatory cells and mucus secreting connective tissue.

539 Stretch and strap for six weeks. At six weeks, if heel not neutral and foot not plantigrade, operate.

Surgery: posteromedial release
- i) elongate tendo Achilles
- ii) capsulotomy of ankle and subtalar joints
- iii) divide inferior tibio-fibular ligament
- iv) divide all tight medial ligaments and capsules

Followed by POP in overcorrected position for six weeks; then D.B. bootees and stretching. Late cases may need bony surgery.

540 It frequently presents with a non-specific picture, indistinguishable from benign biliary disease which thus delays early diagnosis and curative treatment.
It metastasises early both directly to the liver bed and also along the lymphatics.

541 They can protrude both below the chin and upward into the mouth. Excision should be through a submental incision.

542 Dilating oesophageal strictures. They are passed down over guide wires which can be introduced under endoscopic control.

543 Hepatic vein obstruction; Most commonly due to neoplastic encroachment from local tissue, more rarely due to congenital obstruction or thrombosis. Bush-Tea drinking in adults may cause it, or other causes of veno-occlusive disease.

544 No. Thyroid tissue is always midline. Any tissue of thyroid origin found laterally is metastatic and in most cases will be examples of papillary carcinoma.

545 a) Postural - often in adolescents and pregnant women.
b) Muscle weakness - in polio and muscular dystrophies.
c) Compensatory - C.D.H.

546 Of what injury is this recommended?:- "If there is even slight displacement, open reduction and internal fixation are mandatory, because this is the one site in children in which non-union is likely, and if mal-union occurs the result is progressive cubitus valgus during subsequent growth, and the development of ulnar palsy"

547 What types of stimulation of the detrusor muscle of the bladder may lead to a 'contracted bladder'?

548 The antibiotic treatment of chronic prostatitis is often unsuccessful. What reason is usually advanced to explain this?

549 The duodenum can be obstructed from congenital bands, webs or diaphragm. What pancreatic anomaly can cause duodenal obstruction?

550 May a paracolostomy hernia be adequately controlled by wearing a belt?

551 Which part of the brachial plexus lies behind the scalenus anterior muscle?

552 What instructions should be given to a patient who is going to start a course of carbimazole for hyperthyroidism?

553 Give six clinico-pathological types of solitary thyroid nodule.

546 Fracture of the lateral condyle of the humerus = capitellar fracture.

547 Infection (Non-specific acute/chronic; T.B.; Bilharzia)
Interstitial cystitis
Radiotherapy
Chemicals
Carcinoma
Spinal cord damage (e.g. Spina bifida; traumatic paraplegia; multiple sclerosis)

548 The infection may either be in the prostatic tissue or the prostatic fluid. Many antibiotics cannot cross the prostatic epithelium to reach the fluid.

549 An annular pancreas.

550 Usually not.

551 The roots and the trunks emerge from its lateral border, to cross the posterior triangle of the neck.

552 That it must be taken 8-hourly not 'three times a day'. A common cause of treatment failure can be attributed to irregular timing of the drug. The most important and rare side effect is bone marrow depression which is unrelated to dosage or length of treatment. Thus warn them to report any sore throat to their doctor or you. (Sore throat is a common presentation of leucopenia.) Minor side effects usually occur in the first eight weeks.

553 Toxic adenoma
Active follicular adenoma
Inactive follicular disease
Simple nodule
Follicular carcinoma
Papillary carcinoma

554 What are the two commonest complications of prolonged endotracheal intubation in children and how can they be avoided?

555 What is the usual duration of fibrinolytic therapy such as streptokinase?

556 What further treatment can you offer a patient with advanced carcinoma of the prostate unresponsive to oestrogens?

557 For whom might you order an elemental diet?

558 What criteria have been used for deciding which kidney to operate upon first in a case of bilateral renal calculus? What is the currently recognised order?

559 In which age group is mammography least helpful in diagnosis of breast carcinoma and why?

560 How and where is a tibial traction pin placed?

554 1) Blockage of the tube. Regular suction with the instillation of saline down the tube.

2) Subglottic stenosis. Provided a small enough tube is inserted always to allow an air leak around the tube, subglottic stenosis will not occur.

555 72 hours.

556 Irradiation to metastases.
Local resection for urinary obstruction.
Cytotoxic chemotherapy.
Hypophysectomy for bone pain.
(Orchidectomy is of no use, O'Donoghue)

557 Patients with: ulcerative colitis or Crohn's, severe burns, massive small bowel or large bowel resections, major oral or dental surgery, liver disease where precision dieting is vital, and with gastro-intestinal fistulae. Elemental diets may also be used where very low residue is needed pre-operatively as a bowel prep.

558 The size of the respective calculi, the quality of renal function as judged by I.V.U. or differential catheterisation (ureteric) or renography (the best). Badenoch recommended operating on the side with the greater obstruction to stimulate that kidney when the better one was operated upon subsequently. Sreenevasan, in a large series, operated first on the better side as determined by renogram. In calculous anuria, renography was done as soon as rehydration/dialysis were completed, and retrograde pyelography was avoided. *(Annals R.C.S. Eng. 1974, 55.)*

559 The young nulliparous woman, because the breast shows as a homogenous density and it is difficult to distinguish the shadow of a mass. After the menopause the glandular tissue atrophies and mammograms are easier to interpret.

560 1 cm below the tibial tubercle inserted from the lateral side (this approach allows for the asymmetrical shape of the tibia and is far easier).

561 How would you treat a post-operative subphrenic abscess?

562 Patients with active ulcerative colitis may have areas of inflammatory, pseudopolypoid and relatively normal flat mucosa. In which type of mucosa is the pre-cancerous change thought to occur?

563 To be effective lumbar sympathectomy divides which type of nerve fibre?

564 What does this arteriogram report describe? "The main arteries are perfectly smooth and normal as far as the knee or elbow, and there are points of occlusion clear and sharp without proximal irregularity, but without any patent segment beyond the block. A fine complex of root like collaterals spring from the lower end of the patent part of the main artery but does not re-enter below".

565 Which physical signs distinguish a saphena varix from a femoral hernia?

566 What different aspects of gastric function are measured by: pentagastrin, histamine, and insulin tests?

567 What eponym attaches to interstitial cystitis?

561 This is controversial and management has changed over the last decade. Previously subphrenic abscesses were drained early, nowadays they tend to be drained late.

Decide whether there is an underlying cause that requires its own remedy (e.g. biliary fistula); if not, and usually there is none, manage conservatively with high doses of appropriate antibiotics. The vast majority resolve spontaneously or discharge through the original wound. If the patient continues to be toxic and unwell or if the antibiotics do not seem to be aiding resolution, formal drainage may become necessary.

562 The flat mucosa rather than the inflammatory or pseudo-polypoid. *(Leonard Jones et al. Gastroenterology (1977) 73 1280-1289.)*

563 The in-transit pre-ganglionic fibres to blood vessels which synapse in the sacral ganglia.

564 Buerger's disease.

565 These two are surprisingly easy to confuse. Both may be "reducible", have a cough impulse and may disappear on lying down. A fluid thrill will be transmitted to the saphena varix by tapping the saphenous vein in the erect position. Pressing in the groin above the varix when supine abolishes it on standing. Neither of these two signs can be elicited with a femoral hernia.

566 Pentagastrin and histamine tests estimate the total functioning parietal cell mass, whereas the insulin test assesses the vagally induced acidity.

567 Hunner of Hunner's Ulcer. *(G.L. Hunner 1868-1951, Johns Hopkins University U.S.A.)*

568 Which type of malignant thyroid tumour is commoner in areas of endemic goitre?

569 What are the named arteries supplying the stomach?

570 Which endocrine glands are involved in the familial condition of multiple endocrine adenomatosis type 1?

571 What are the basic changes in the anatomy of the gastro-oesophageal junction that surgery sets out to achieve in order to control reflux?

572 What types of laboratory investigation are carried out on a segment of bowel affected by Hirschsprung's disease?

573 If megavoltage irradiation of a bladder tumour fails to control it what should then be done?

574 What is the commonest cause of a renal mass in neonates?

575 What are the different cell types found in the parathyroid gland?

568 The follicular type.

569 The stomach has a profuse blood supply:
Left gastric ....from the coeliac
Right gastric ......from the common hepatic
Gastroduodenal .....from the common hepatic
Short gastric (vasa brevia) .....from the splenic
Left gastroepiploic .....from the splenic
Right gastroepiploic .... from the gastroduodenal

570 Parathyroid, pituitary, pancreas, adrenal cortex.

571 If the oesophagus is effectively shortened by pathology it can be lengthened by fashioning part of the stomach into a tube thereby making the lower end of the new oesophagus intra-abdominal. Alternatively, if the valvular mechanism is at fault the oesophagus can be drawn down and fixed and or stomach drawn around it to form a one way valve system with the lower end of the oesophagus again intra-abdominal. If gastric acid be high, a vagotomy may be helpful, and a gastric drainage procedure may be needed in addition.

572 a) Quantitative cholinesterase activity. (Increased in the affected segment.)
b) Histology. (Hypertrophic nerve fibres and absent ganglion cells.)
c) Histochemistry. (To establish rapid frozen section estimation of the extent of the disease at operation.)

573 This is controversial: If the patient is sufficiently fit, total cystectomy with urinary diversion may be undertaken. N.B. Salvage cystectomy after a full course of D.X.T. carries a high morbidity. Most surgeons prefer to allow several months to elapse from the time of limited irradiation (2000Rads - 4000Rads). In unfit patients symptomatic treatment must suffice.

574 Hydronephrosis from pelvi-ureteric stenosis. (Second commonest is multicystic kidney).

575 Principal cells, water-clear cells, and oxyphil cells.

576 The continuous irrigation method of pre-operative bowel preparation using a balanced electrolytic solution with added neomycin via naso-gastric tube with the patient on a cholera table has what main disadvantages?

577 What are the bony deformities found in a supracondylar fracture of the humerus?

578 In intestinal obstruction how reliable are the symptoms and signs of strangulation as an indicator of bowel viability?

579 What is the action of metoclopramide (Maxolon)?

580 What is a mulberry stone?

581 How many calyces are there in each kidney as seen on I.V.U.?

576 Although it achieves mechanical clearance of the bowel in three to four hours and eliminates E.Coli and most of the other large bowel flora, it fails to eliminate bacteroides and, of course, is contraindicated in obstruction of the bowel.

577 The distal fragment is posteriorly displaced
internally rotated
angulated transversely
proximally displaced.

578 Pain: unreliable. (It may be severe without strangulation although a steady severe pain is in favour of strangulation.)

Tenderness: not universal. (About 20% of strangulated cases show no tenderness.)

Temperature: useful. (It is more commonly raised in strangulation than non-strangulated cases.)

Pulse: as an initial measure not very useful, but a steady or sudden rise may be highly significant.

Leucocytosis: again not very helpful, although a high W.B.C. supports a diagnosis of strangulation.

Distension of the abdomen: not helpful.

Sudden onset of symptoms: favours strangulation.

Shock: may well be septicaemic and occur early in strangulation, but rarely is due to dehydration in non-strangulated cases.

579 a) Cerebral: depression of the vomiting centre.
b) Abdominal: it has a direct effect on gastric smooth muscle and regulates gastric and duodenal contraction. This action is not affected by vagotomy.

580 A calcium oxalate calculus. This type of stone is covered with sharp projections that cause local bleeding giving the stone its characteristic speckled appearance.

581 7 in all. Upper pole 3, middle 2, lower pole 2.

582 There are three main groups of glands in the prostate. Which is associated with benign hypertrophy, and which with carcinoma?

583 What dose of radiation is given by a screening mammogram and what sort of criteria are used in the selection of patients likely to benefit from a mammography screening programme?

584 What are the contraindications to extraperitoneal tunnelling of a terminal colostomy?

585 A lumbar hernia usually protrudes through the triangle of Petit (formed by iliac crest, lat. dorsi, and ext. oblique). What is the differential diagnosis?

586 List the differential diagnosis of a child presenting with a painful hip.

587 Briefly describe the anterior compartment syndrome.

582 (i) Mucosal, opening directly into the urethra.
(ii) Submucosal or periurethral which are the glands that enlarge in benign prostatic hypertrophy.
(iii) Outer glands or the main prostatic glands which produce most of the prostatic secretions and which are the site of most prostatic carcinomata.

583 Dosages vary according to apparatus used, techniques employed, number of films taken, and views required. The Manchester service has reduced their dosage range to approximately 0.2 Rads. Long term studies of therapeutic/accidental radiation induced breast cancer indicate the increased risk of cancer after a latent period of 20 years. Thus repeated mammography should probably be limited to high risk patients over 35 years, and normal risk patients over 50 years. *(Leader B.M.J. (1977) 1 191-192)*

584 A short fat-laden mesentery as is often found in obese patients.
A short length of bowel is available to tunnel.

585 A cold abscess.
A phantom hernia due to local muscular paresis. This can be suprisingly difficult to diagnose unless you think of it.

586 Infection: bone or joint
Trauma
Tumour: osteogenic sarcoma
Irritable hip
Perthe's disease
Slipped upper femoral epiphysis
Missed CDH (although this is usually painless)

587 Oedema of muscles of the anterior fascial compartment of the(lower) leg (enclosed by tibia, interosseous ligament and fibula) is caused by excessive exercise or trauma - especially fractured tib./fib., or by arterial embolism or thrombosis. It results in pain, tenderness and a woody hard swelling in the anterior leg and leads to ischaemic necrosis of muscles, anterior tibial artery thrombosis, anterior tibial nerve necrosis, and contracture of the muscles which may eventually be overcome by gravity to leave a foot drop and impaired walking.

588 What are the common causes of post-operative mortality following total or subtotal gastrectomy for cancer apart from the cancer itself?

589 Name a rare, but possibly fatal complication peculiar to highly selective (or proximal) vagotomy

590 What are the important differential diagnoses of a rectal prolapse in a child?

591 Name some of the important features of an acute rejection episode in a renal transplant patient.

592 List the different possible types of portal decompressive procedures.

593 You are shown a pot of a child's kidney with obvious tumour in it accompanied by a bone containing metastases. Which is more likely, nephroblastoma (Wilm's) or neuroblastoma?

594 What are the contraindications to barium enema reduction of an intussusception?

595 In terms of the timing of its appearance, which cases of jaundice in the newborn need to be fully investigated?

588 Leaking from the anastomosis.
Respiratory complications.
General complications associated with major operations (e.g. pulmonary emboli).

589 Lesser curve necrosis.

590 Rectal polyp; intussusception; (haemorrhoids rare).

591 Decrease in urinary output, urinary (urea) and sodium content, and a fall in urine osmolarity and creatinine clearance. There may be renal tenderness and swelling, pyrexia, tachycardia. Casts and mononuclear cells may be seen in the urine.

592 End to side porta-caval anastomosis
Side to side " " "
Side to side " " dacron H-graft
End to side spleno-renal anastomosis
Side to side " " "
Distal spleno-renal shunt (with division of L gastric/ coronary veins, R gastro-epiploics((Women)
Mesentero-caval dacron H-graft

593 Neuroblastoma.

594 a) An ill or shocked child even after satisfactory resuscitation.
b) Radiological evidence of acute obstruction i.e. dilated loops of small bowel with fluid level.
c) Possibly those over two years or cases twice recurrent since there is a greater likelihood of there being a significant lesion at the apex.

595 Those in which the jaundice appears in the first 24 hours after birth, and those in which jaundice persists for more than a week after birth.

596 What percentage of patients with carcinoma of the hypopharynx and post-cricoid region have involved nodes at the time of presentation?

597 What is the cause of pain in the few cases of this type?

598 How else may such a tumour present?

599 What are the indications for surgery in chronic pancreatitis?

600 Name some of the causes of duodenal stump leakage.

601 What are the causes of hypercalciuria?

602 Discuss the management of a patient in her third trimester of pregnancy who complains of severe colicky central and lower abdominal pain.

603 A small % of patients presenting with urinary retention in fact have chronic retention with a high blood urea level. Standard treatment consists of catheter drainage until the urea falls to normal or stabilises. What metabolic disturbance often accompanies this period?

596 50% overall. 75% in patients with carcinoma of the pyriform fossa.

597 Referred otalgia from the glosso-pharyngeal nerve (tympanic branch = Jacobsen's nerve).

598 Weight loss, dysphonia, sore throat, dry throat, pneumonia from aspiration, recurrent laryngeal nerve palsy, haemorrhage.

599 a) Pain uncontrolled by ordinary analgesics.
b) Repeated attacks of acute pancreatitis.
c) Complications: cyst/fistula/portal vein obstruction.
d) Doubtful diagnosis - (carcinoma?).

600 a) Poor suturing technique.
b) Excessive mobilisation of the stump which may imperil the blood supply.
c) Obstruction to the afferent loop.
d) Gross malnutrition - anaemia, hypoproteinaemia, lack of vitamins etc.

601 Idiopathic hypercalciuria (by far the commonest cause).
Hypercalcaemia.
Primary hyperparathyroidism.
Renal tubular acidosis.
Immobilisation.
Paget's disease.
Vitamin D overdose.
Neoplasm.

602 Colicky central lower abdominal pain in the third trimester is almost always uterine. The differential diagnosis includes labour, abruptio placentae, red degeneration in a fibroid. Rarely pain may be caused by a urinary tract infection or constipation. An obstetrician must be consulted immediately.

603 Sodium chloride depletion. It is essential to provide adequate fluid and electrolyte replacement by IV route. Closely monitor plasma and urinary electrolyte levels.

604 Partial cystectomy for cancer is done very infrequently nowadays. Why is this?

605 What are the essential prerequisites to the safe transfer of surgical neonates from one hospital to another, and how would you recommend they be instituted?

606 Give an outline classification of the causes of intestinal obstruction.

607 What are the causes of joint stiffness following injury?

608 Apparent total destruction of a joint due to septic arthritis in an infant as diagnosed on X-ray may be deceptive. Why?

609 What is the management of hydrocele in children?

604 The lesion must be single, have a sharp margin, and the rest of the bladder must be normal. Excision should allow at least a 2 cm margin of excision. These conditions seldom obtain. Implantation of the tumour in the wound scar is a rare but well recognised complication which leads to lingering morbidity.

605 (i) Warmth - use silver foil and Gamgee. Portable incubator if possible.

(ii) Empty stomach particularly in intestinal obstruction. Pass nasogastric tube and aspirate quarter-hourly.

(iii) Maintain airway and adequate oxygenation.

(iv) A good paediatric nurse.

606 Mechanical: From outside the bowel: hernia, volvulus, adhesions, intussusception etc.
From the wall itself: carcinoma, stricture, Crohn's.
Luminal: impacted stone, polyp, F.B.etc.

Neurogenic: ileus, drugs etc.

Vascular: thrombosis/embolus etc.

607 Common: Fractures into joints
Severe soft tissue injuries around joints
Prolonged immobilisation of joints following injury

Uncommon: Myositis
Sudeks
Late O.A.
Crossunion
Infection
Missed dislocation

608 Inflammation can cause such decalcification as to make an infant bone radiotranslucent. Arthrography will show up an intact joint.

609 No action is required in infants as about 90% resolve by one year. Persistent hydroceles should be operated upon by school age.

610 What are the main complications of an ileostomy fashioned for a patient who has had a pan-proctocolectomy for ulcerative colitis?

611 Is carcinoma of the colon commoner in men or women?

612 Describe a Z-plasty.

613 Define erosive gastritis.

614 With what conditions is erosive gastritis associated, or of what may it be a complication?

610 Immediate
Gangrene of an ischaemic spout; Infection, Dermatitis; Psychiatric; Haemorrhage (major or minor).

Early
Difficulty in managing the bag - especially in blind/handicapped patients; difficulty in dietary control; dehydration due to even minor degrees of gastroenteritis; dermatitis around the ileostomy - usually a question of careful siting and then fashioning the stoma and nursing care later.

Late
Prolapse of the ileostomy; Obstruction (which can be due to kinking of the terminal ileum by adhesions or small bowel herniating into the lateral space, if not closed); Urinary calculi.

611 Women. *(6:4 Reg. Gen. in England 1973 Annual Report.)* (Men have a higher incidence of Ca. rectum.)

612 A Z-plasty is a common manoeuvre beloved of plastic surgeons that consists of forming two triangular transposition flaps whose common edge lies along the line of tissue tension or pull that is then relieved or lengthened by the transposition of those flaps. The angle formed at the apex of the triangular flap i.e. the angle of the arms of the Z, will determine the increase in length achieved. An angle of 60° will produce up to 75% increase in the distance between the original apices of the flaps (at the expense of increased lateral tension).

613 Erosive gastritis is a diffuse lesion of the gastric mucosa characterised by multiple acute ulcers within the lamina propria found only in the parietal cell bearing area. (The antrum is rarely involved.) *(Reynolds, Annals R.C.S. (1974) 55 213-225.)*

614 Steroid/Aspirin/Alcohol ingestion or administration.
Head injury.
Burns.
Gross sepsis.
Shock.
Major trauma or major injury.

615 Why may erosive gastritis be such a dangerous condition?

616 In what way does the management of 'gastroschisis' differ from that of exomphalos?

617 What is the prognosis of sacrococcygeal tumour?

618 What does this describe:- 'A battleground between macrophages and indigestible antigen.'

619 Is the foramen of Bochdalek situated at the front or back of the diaphragm?

620 Describe the management of the clinically solitary thyroid nodule.

621 Gall stone colic typically occurs at night. What is the explanation usually advanced for this?

622 What structures lie immediately behind the first part of the duodenum?

615 Haemorrhage may be severe and continuous even after major surgery which carries a high mortality. The surgery may be vagotomy and drainage, Polya gastrectomy or Billroth I partial gastrectomy, the latter carrying the lowest mortality rate. (Bile which exacerbates the condition is least likely to regurgitate back into the stomach after a Billroth I than other procedures.) *(Reynolds, Annals R.C.S. Eng. (1974) 55 213-225.)*

616 It presents a surgical emergency as peritonitis may develop and lead to septicaemia. Frequently repair can be achieved by primary closure.

617 These lesions are rarely malignant in infancy (less than 10%) but if left untreated may become malignant.

618 A granuloma. (These can be divided into high and low turnover for instance sarcoid/T.B./Crohn's/primary biliary cirrhosis cause high turnover granulomata, whereas carbon material would cause a low turnover granuloma. High turnover is characterised by epithelioid and giant cells.

619 Back.

620 a) History and examination.
b) Thyroid function tests.
c) Thyroid scan.
d) Operative preparations where indicated (view cords etc.).

All non-functioning (cold) nodules should be removed by partial thyroidectomy.
Most functioning nodules should also be removed because only in this way can the true nature of the lesion be proved.
Some functioning nodules in older or poor risk patients may be suitable for radioactive iodine therapy.

621 It is thought to be due to the position of the patient. The stones tend to congregate at the neck of the gall bladder when the patient lies flat.

622 Portal vein, common bile duct, gastro-duodenal artery.

623 What investigations should you perform for recurrent pain after ulcer surgery?

624 A very severe first attack, disease affecting the whole colon, advanced age of the patient, are all ominous features of ulcerative colitis. How common is the acute fulminant form of ulcerative colitis?

625 What is gastroschisis? (N.B. It occurs most often in the premature, male infant on the right side and is often accompanied by small bowel atresia.)

626 Intercostal drainage of an acute empyema when necessary is achieved by tube drainage; this gives an airtight wound allowing suction and prevents entry or air into the pleural cavity. What are the problems of this method?

627 What differentiates a paralytic ileus from secondary mechanical obstruction?

628 What are the important symptoms of acute prostatitis?

629 Following removal of a large gall stone obstructing the ileum what should be done to the gall bladder at that same operation?

630 How may a pre-operative diagnosis of hepatic hydatid cyst be confirmed?

623 Repeat history and physical examination in case the initial diagnosis was faulty.
Fibre-optic endoscopy with biopsy if indicated.
Serum gastrin level.
Acid secretion studies using insulin and pentagastrin.
Barium meal and follow through.
Cholecystogram if endoscopy and barium studies are negative.

624 About 5% *(Bailey and Love.)*

625 The failure of completion of one or other lateral fold of somatopleure forming the abdominal wall. Any part of the gut can prolapse into it and no sac covers it. It is situated lateral to the umbilicus distinguishing it from an omphalocoele.

626 Pain. Blockage of the tube. Failure to achieve adequate drainage. Tube falling out.

627 The patient with paralytic ileus has no colic, absent or tinkling bowel sounds and X-ray may show fluid levels in both large and small bowel.

628 Pyrexia, malaise ± rigors. Concomitant or delayed urinary tract symptoms of frequency and difficulty in micturition sometimes progress to retention of urine. Rectal pain, perineal discomfort, backache, and tenesmus may also occur.

629 Nothing.

630 By serology.
(Casoni skin reagent is no longer available.)

631 Scattered calcification in both kidneys in the distribution of the calyceal pattern may be seen in which conditions on plain X-ray?

632 How significant is pain in regard to carcinoma of the oesophagus?

633 The treatment of impacted calculi in the submandibular gland is usually excision of the gland. Where do they usually impact?

634 What is the difference between the natural histories of intermittent claudication due to aorto-iliac disease and that due to femoro-popliteal disease? Are the results of arterial reconstruction equally good in the two groups?

635 List some of the common clinical conditions associated with an increased risk of infection.

636 What is Well's operation for rectal prolapse?

637 What type of bone pain does a malignant tumour of bone typically produce?

638 What are the grounds for arguing that total thyroidectomy may be the correct treatment for both follicular and papillary carcinoma of the thyroid?

631 Nephrocalcinosis of hypercalcaemia, e.g. hyperparathyroidism.
Medullary sponge kidneys.
Renal tubular acidosis.

632 It is usually a late feature but by itself is not a contraindication to an exploratory operation.

633 a) The hilum of the gland just below the lingual nerve.
b) The posterior part of the extraglandular duct where it is crossed by the lingual nerve.
note: c) If the calculus impacts in the distal duct, it can be removed through the mouth with a simple small procedure.

634 Aorto-iliac: generally slower in onset and progression but there is a lower incidence of spontaneous recovery than with femoro-popliteal.

Femoro-popliteal: occlusions naturally improve and stabilise and after 5 years only approximately 5-10% progress.

The results of femoro-popliteal grafts are less good than of aorto-iliac.

635 Diabetes mellitus.
Corticosteroids.
Thermal injury.
Alcoholism.
Protein or calorie malnutrition.
Foreign bodies in the tissues.
Arteriosclerosis.
Neutropenia due to marrow depression.

636 The insertion of a plastic foam sheet (Ivalon sponge) stitched around the rectum and to the sacrum to create adhesions which pull the rectum back up into the abdomen.

637 Constant rather than transient, and worse at night.

638 Papillary carcinomata are often multifocal and thus partial thyroidectomy may leave some tumour behind. Total thyroidectomy is indicated in follicular carcinoma if there is distant metastasis necessitating treatment by *131 Iodine.

639 Describe a gumma.

640 Calcification of the vas deferens may be seen on X-ray. What can cause it?

641 List the commoner complications of appendicectomy.

642 Why does carcinoma of the hypopharynx and post-cricoid carcinoma usually present late?

643 Where are the lymph nodes of Gerota?

644 Which organisms commonly cause osteomyelitis in a child of 6 years? Which antibiotics are useful?

645 Where is the bowel said to distend most in a large bowel obstruction?

639 A gumma is the classical focal lesion of tertiary syphilis; usually solitary, consisting of coagulative necrosis similar to caseation but retaining more of the architecture. It is surrounded by a zone of lymphocytes, plasma cells and macrophages, fibroblasts and fibrous tissue. Adjacent arteries show endarteritis obliterans.

640 Unilaterally - T.B. Bilaterally - Diabetes mellitus.

641 Early

General: Chest infection
Urinary retention
Septicaemia
Pulmonary embolus (D.V.T.)

Local: Haemorrhage (Primary, Reactionary, Secondary.)
Infection:- Intraperitoneal
Extraperitoneal - wound infection
Abscess formation
Adhesions - small bowel obstruction
Fistulae - think of Crohn's

Late

Adhesions
Incisional hernia
Right inguinal hernia

642 The patient frequently ignores early symptoms of mild dysphagia.

643 Pararectal, lying just above levator ani close to the rectal wall in the region of the ampulla.

644 Staph. aureus: Flucloxacillin, cloxacillin, penicillin, fusidic acid, clindamycin.
Strep. Group A: Benzyl penicillin.
Haemophilus influ. type B: chloramphenicol, ampicillin co-trimoxazole (Septrin).

645 At the caecum. Thus caecal tenderness may be an indication for urgent surgery to forestall perforation and general peritonitis.

646 Frusemide in high dosage may be the cause of which abdominal condition?

647 What complication (pre or post-operative) of surgery for carcinoma of the lung or bronchus may improve the prognosis?

648 What are the main indications for adenoidectomy?

649 What are the main principles that justify the use of regional isolated limb perfusion for malignancy?

650 One of those terribly big questions that you occasionally get asked is 'Discuss the management of hand injuries'. What categories of injury should you include? N.B. In each category you would discuss the relevance of the different structures - skin,tendon, muscle, nerve, bone, etc., and it would be wise to make a separate item of general principles of treatment in for instance control of oedema/stiffness/infection, which is common to all hand injuries.

651 Describe the basic steps in the operative treatment of sigmoid volvulus, in the likely absence of ileal involvement? Ref. *B.J.H.M. 1976 (Jan.).*

646 Acute pancreatitis.

647 Infection. Controlled intra-pleural infection with B.C.G. has been shown to improve the prognosis after lung cancer surgery. *(McKneally et al, Lancet (1976) 1 377-379.)*

648 1. seromucinous otitis media ("glue ear").
2. persistent nasal obstruction and rhinorrhoea.
3. recurrent upper respiratory tract infections, including sinusitis.
4. postural apnoea (total obstruction of upper airway by enlarged adenoids and tonsils).

649 Higher concentrations of cytotoxic agents may be delivered to the tumour than by the systemic route.
Cells in transit between primary site and the regional lymph nodes may be killed.
Malignant cells left behind or 'Locked In' after regional node block dissection may be killed.

650 Lacerations - clean/dirty superficial/deep.
Fractures/dislocations.
Crushing injuries.
Degloving injuries.
Burns - thermal/chemical/radiation.
Bullet wound injuries - high/low velocity single/multiple.
Foreign body penetration - splinters/grease gun injuries.
Loss of digits.

651 Incision: left oblique or right paramedian, (reserve left paramedian for closure of Hartmann procedure). Decompress the large bowel loop and deliver the volvulus into the wound. If the bowel is not gangrenous, untwist it and either clamp off redundant bowel and carry out sigmoidectomy with end to end anastomosis or perform sigmoid mesenteropexy. If the bowel is overtly gangrenous avoid untwisting it, to prevent systemic escape of toxins but place clamps on proximal and distal bowel and mesentery. Resect bowel and carry out either a primary end to end anastomosis or Hartmann procedure if the ends fail to meet without a lot of mobilisation.

652 Perforation of the gall bladder, or bile ducts causes free bile in the peritoneal cavity: may this occur in other conditions?

653 Name some of the causes of urethral diverticula (in men).

654 When is portal venography contraindicated?

655 What are the findings on bimanual examination of the bladder (which must be done under G.A. with muscle relaxation), which will decide the extent of tumour on the T.N.M. classification?

656 Why is appendicitis in children under 5 years old so serious?

657 What have dental extraction, urethral instrumentation, barium enema and sigmoidoscopy in common?

658 When does cystic hygroma usually present and where?

659 What percentage of clinically solitary thyroid nodules are malignant?

652 Yes. Perforated peptic ulcer (generally duodenal).
Primary biliary peritonitis.

653 Congenital.
Raised pressure due to stricture.
Persistent calculus (stuck in the urethra).
An in-dewlling catheter (especially in paraplegics).
Iatrogenic (a false passage- after urethroplasty).

654 Prothrombin time over 15 sec.
Platelet count under 100,000.
Deep jaundice.

655 T_1 A soft mass, mobile within the bladder without evidence of infiltration (i.e. generally impalpable).
T_2 A thickened indurated wall but not hard, not nodular.
T_3 A hard mass but mobile.
T_4 A mass fixed to the pelvis or tethered so that mobility is impaired in one or other direction or a mass infiltrating the vagina or prostate.

656 Because most cases are perforated by the time they are seen at hospital. There is frequently a delay in appreciation of the symptoms and localisation of intra-peritoneal infection is less effective. Fluid deprivation and losses are more serious in children.

657 They may all cause a transient bacteraemia. Gram-negative bacilli are less likely to lodge in the crevices of an endocardial valve than the Streptococci commonly found on blood culture after dentistry, or the faecal Strep. after anal or urethral instrumentation.

658 In the lower 1/3 neck, posterior triangle of an infant.

659 About 50% of clinically solitary nodules are found at operation not to be solitary.
About 25% of truly solitary nodules are carcinomatous, thus about 12% of clinically solitary nodules are carcinomatous.

660 What are the various possible methods of urinary diversion?

661 What indicates non-union of a fracture?

662 How do you distinguish between the cut end of a ureter and a cut artery that has stopped bleeding?

663 Describe the important stages of a left hemicolectomy.

664 How long does it take a bacteriologist to identify an anaerobic Gram-negative septicaemic from the time he receives the blood culture specimen?

665 Apart from torsion, haematocele or haematoma and epididymo-orchitis, what other conditions of non-infective and non-traumatic origin may cause an acutely swollen and tender scrotum?

660 Kidney level: nephrostomy, pyelostomy, ileal conduit to skin or bladder.
Ureteric level: cutaneous ureterostomy, ureterosigmoid-ostomy, trigone colostoplasty, rectal bladder and proximal colostomy, rectal bladder and intersphincteric colostomy, ileal or colonic conduit.
Bladder level: suprapubic cystostomy, cutaneous vesicostomy, suprapubic displacement of the urethra.
Urethral level: perineal urethrostomy, urethral catheter.

661 Possible deformity.
Mobility in the absence of tenderness.
Radiologically the fracture persists often without evidence of callus formation and the bone ends are sclerotic and rounded.

662 The ureter pouts at its end, the adjacent part vermiculates on gentle stimulation, whereas an arterial lumen contracts further.

663 X-match 2 units of blood. Prep. the bowel. Use nasogastric tube and urinary catheter, ± subcutaneous heparin or other acceptable prophylaxis against D.V.T. General anaesthesia. Skin prep. Drapes etc. Through a left paramedian or midline incision first make a thorough abdominal exploration for metastatic disease. Dissect from laterally, identify and the preserve the left ureter. Perform a high ligation of the inferior mesenteric vein and artery. Mobilise the splenic flexure and divide the transverse colon yet retaining the middle colic artery to preserve the arterial supply to the proximal end of the anastomosis. Resect the left side of the colon down to lower sigmoid and perform primary anastomosis with covering colostomy or double-barrelled colostomy for later closure.

664 At least 48 hours, and often as long as three days. Anaerobic bacteria (e.g. Bacteroides) grow very slowly in culture.

665 Testicular tumours.
Idiopathic fat necrosis.
Idiopathic scrotal oedema (testicle feels normal).

666 What may mimic a renal calculus on a plain X-ray?

667 On a lymphangiogram is it usual to see the lymph glands along the internal iliac artery outlined?

668 What are the possible skin manifestations of impaired lymphatic drainage?

669 Define varicocele.

670 Are there any blood tests which are really helpful in confirming a clinical diagnosis of fat embolism?

671 Which cell type predominates in parathyroid hyperplasia?

672 What is the danger of using the umbilical vein as a route of choice for giving intravenous fluids?

673 If a varicocele appeared on the left side suddenly in a middle aged man, what should you do?

674 What is the incidence of non-union in the conservative management of intra-capsular femoral neck fracture?

675 Which type of thyroid carcinoma may be multifocal?

666 Calcified lymph nodes.
Gall stones.
Ingested pills.
Phleboliths.
Chip fracture of L.1.
Calcified adrenal gland.
Calcified old T.B. in the kidney.
Ossified tip of 12th rib.

667 No - such appearances suggest lymphatic obstruction which produces retrograde flow and collateral channel filling. Equally one does not normally see the mesenteric lymph nodes outlined.

668 Lymphoedema.
Eczema.
Dermatitis.
Cellulitis.
Hyperkeratosis.
Papillomatosis.

669 Varicosity of the internal spermatic vein ± the cremasteric veins.

670 Not really. D.I.C. often accompanies severe fat embolism, and blood tests may indicate the presence of the former.

671 The clear cell.

672 There is a proven association between umbilical vein catheterisation and necrotising enterocolitis. The umbilicus is often infected and this may predispose to septicaemia and portal vein thrombosis.

673 Examine the patient thoroughly and perform an I.V.U. looking for possible obstruction to the left renal vein.

674 Between 30-40%.

675 Papillary.

676 If a patient with a stricture of the membranous urethra requires a prostatectomy, to what special risk is he subject?

677 What are the indications for choledochoduodenostomy?

678 What suture material should be used to close the lateral space in a left iliac colostomy?

679 What vertebral body deformity always accompanies lateral curvature in a fixed scoliosis?

680 What is the incidence of asymptomatic gall stones in autopsies of people over 50 years?

681 What % of people found to have gall stones as seen on plain X-ray are going to develop symptoms at some time?

682 What are the indications for a cervical sympathectomy?

683 What are the usual symptoms of a para-oesophageal hernia?

684 What structure should be protected in dividing the strap muscles in a partial thyroidectomy operation?

685 Why may gall stone colic be felt in the left hypochondrium?

676 Post-operative incontinence, because the external sphincter is often already damaged in these cases.

677 Controversial: some surgeons say that you should seldom do it; many employ it when the common bile duct contains multiple or recurrent stones with or without stricture at its lower end.

678 It should be non-absorbable to discourage the gutter from re-forming, thus preventing entrapment of small bowel between colon and parietal wall.

679 Rotation of the vertebral bodies towards the concave side.

680 Approximately 10%. *(Bateson and Bouchier B.M.J. 1975 4 427-429).*

681 Figures vary but 50% is commonly quoted (See reference above).

682 Primary or secondary Raynaud's disease with nutritional loss.
Arterial occlusion in the subclavian or brachial vessels.
Severe hyperhidrosis.
Causalgia.
Phantom limb pains } if chemical block with marcaine is shown to be effective first
Erythrocyanosis.

683 Usually few: oesophagitis or perioesophagitis is absent because the sphincter is normal. If the hernia is very large the patient may notice intermittent hiccough, dysphagia and cardiac embarrassment. Recurrent nipping of the neck of the hernia may cause ischaemia of its apex with a developing iron deficiency anaemia.

684 The ansa hypoglossi. The innervation of the strap muscles enters low down therefore divide the strap muscle high up.

685 Embryologically the gall bladder develops as a midline structure and has a bilateral innervation.

686 What are the common predisposing causes of rectal prolapse in children?

687 If you were on a camping holiday miles from civilisation and your son developed a probable torsion of the testicle, which way would you attempt to untwist it?

688 In which variety of hernia is a Richter's type of strangulation found most commonly?

689 Give an outline description of the surgical procedure carried out in the recipient of a renal transplant.

690 The appearance of the cremasteric muscle may give what clues as to the nature of the type of hernia during a hernia repair?

691 Why is vesico-ureteric reflux commoner in children than in adults?

686 Straining at stool in a constipated child.
Diarrhoea as part of a malabsorption syndrome especially cystic fibrosis and coeliac disease.
Explosive or hurried defaecation.
N.B. Uncommon causes include paralysis of the anal sphincters; gross malnutrition; prolapse associated with ectopia vesica.

687 Untwist it in the direction that tends to relieve the pain. Usually the testicles are torted such that from below the left testicle should be untwisted in a clockwise and the right testicle in an anti-clockwise direction. In any case the scrotum should be surgically explored as soon as possible.

688 It is much commoner in femoral that inguinal herniae. It occurs in 0.7% of all femoral herniae, and in 14% of strangulated ones. *(Current surgical diagnosis and treatment. Dunphy & Way; Lange Philadelphia (1975) P.664).*

689 The donor kidney is implanted in the iliac fossa. The major renal vein is anastomosed end to side with the external iliac vein. Other renal veins are ligated. If the donor kidney is from a cadaver, the wall of the aorta with renal artery or arteries is sutured as a patch into the external iliac artery. If the renal artery has no attached aortic patch it is usually sutured end to end with the internal iliac artery. Live donor kidneys with more than two arteries should be anastomosed by the formation of one stoma if possible by the anastomosis of the arteries together. The ureter is taken obliquely through the bladder muscle as an antireflux procedure and anastomosed to mucosa. A Foley catheter is left in the bladder with or without a fine ureteric catheter to drain the pelvis of the donor kidney.

690 An indirect hernia is usually associated with well developed cremaster, but a direct hernia is associated with thin and weak cremaster.

691 It is thought to be due to the shorter length of intramural ureter in the child making a shorter "flap-valve". Intramural distance increases as the child grows older.

692 What are the problems or complications associated with undescended testes?

693 An ectopic testicle most commonly lies in the superficial inguinal pouch. Where else could it lie?

694 Classify urethral stricture.

695 What is the indication for extra-fascial ligation of incompetent perforating veins in the lower leg?

696 What special investigations would you order on a baby or child with suspected Wilm's tumour?

697 Which type of thyroid neoplasms most readily take up iodine?

698 How would you treat a man with a prostatic abscess?

692 Sterility of the affected testis.
Hernia.
Trauma to the testis from its position.
Torsion which is difficult to diagnose.
Malignancy - said to be 35 times the normal risk, but the overall risk is still small, although intra-abdominal testes have higher risk than inguinal ones.

693 It could be perineal, pubic, pubo-penile, femoral, crural, or in the contralateral scrotum.

694 Congenital or acquired.
Inflammatory/infective: GC? TB, following urethral chancre.
Traumatic: External: (usually at membranous part associated with a fractured pelvis, or bulbar part due to 'fall astride' injury).
Internal: Instrumentation; by catheter, endoscope.
Operative; prostatectomy, penis amputation.

695 Extra-fascial ligation is carried out if the perforating veins are incompetent only when the subcutaneous tissues are near-normal i.e. minimal induration, fat necrosis, and fibrosis in the 'gaiter' area. Accurate incision over the perforators is necessary to avoid much lateral dissection which may lead to tissue necrosis. Sub-fascial ligation (Cockett) allows wide dissection.

696 I.V.U. Ultrasound scan. Renal scan if available. Retrograde pyelography used to be performed in the absence of the latter two procedures. N.B. Aortography, venography, and lymphangiography are in most cases unnecessary and hazardous in a child who in all likelihood will have a laparotomy anyway.

697 The follicular type.

698 By draining the abscess, either by T.U.R. or when there is marked peri-prostatic spread, by perineal incision with resultant dependant drainage.

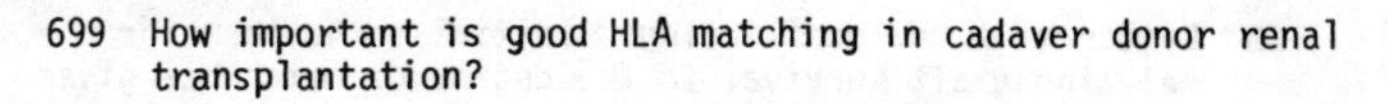

699 How important is good HLA matching in cadaver donor renal transplantation?

700 Name the two benign neoplasms of the kidney.

701 What pre-operative measures should be taken before operating on neonates?

702 What constitute Koch's postulates?

703 What is the advantage of the lateral as opposed to the anterior approach to the adrenal gland?

704 What is the greatest danger of intravenous feeding using a central line and what action should be taken if this is suspected?

705 "In the abdominal type of disease the primary focus in the bowel is so small that it is rarely identifiable, and the manifestation of the infection first is great enlargement of the mesenteric lymph nodes." To what does this refer? What is the old name given to it? In what way does this differ in adults?

706 How should you position a patient for a change of nephrostomy tube?

699 Evidence is now conflicting. Initial enthusiasm for relating graft survival to the degree of match has given way to guarded scepticism of its value. Some complete matches have been followed by rejection. In blood groups A and B, HLA match does seem to correlate with survival, but not for group O. Nevertheless, results of good HLA matching are better than for poor matches. *(Oliver et al, Lancet 1977 2 220.)*

700 Adenoma and angioma.

701 (i) Check that Vit. K_1 has been given.
(ii) Check that the baby's temperature is as near 37° as possible.
(iii) Check that blood has been cross matched.

702 The organism should be found reproducibly in the lesion.
Cultures of the organism must be obtainable from the lesion when grown on artificial media.
Organisms taken from such a culture on an artificial medium should be capable of reproducing the lesion in an animal of the same species as that from which it was isolated.

703 It gives better exposure after resection of the right 10th or 11th left. It suffers from being a unilateral approach in diseases which often affect both adrenals.

704 Septicaemia. A blood culture should be taken and if there is a strong suspicion of septicaemia then the central line should be removed, the tip sent for culture and antibiotics started.

705 Childhood tuberculosis of the gut, clinically "Tabes Mesenterica" which is very different from the adult tuberculous enteritis due to swallowing of infected sputum. The latter leads to circumferential ulcers in the ileum, localised peritonitis, strictures, and fistulae with minimal lymph node involvement.

706 Try and position the patient so that he lies just as he did when it was first inserted.

707 Where is a Spigelian hernia felt?

708 What symptoms suggest an oesophageal atresia and how is the diagnosis made pre-operatively?

709 At operation what should be done in the first instance if a patient with a single kidney has his ureter accidentally ligated or cut?

710 What % of people with gall stones also have common bile duct calculi?

711 What are the uses of balloon-catheter duodenostomy?

712 What are the common complications of such a balloon catheter duodenostomy?

713 Give an outline classification of spinal cord tumours.

707 Lateral to rectus abdominis and usually below the umbilicus.

708 Any baby that is mucousy, salivates a lot or becomes cyanosed after a feed is suggestive of an oesophageal atresia. A firm, size 6 or 8, nasogastric tube is passed and a plain X-ray of chest and abdomen taken. This will show the level of the atresia and whether a lower pouch fistula is present (gas in the bowel).

709 This depends on the skill and experience of the best surgeon available.
If ligated, untie the ligature.
If cut in pelvis, re-implant ureter in bladder +/- psoas hitch or Boari flap.
If cut higher, either attempt re-anastomosis over a ureteric splint, or perform nephrostomy, or both.

710 About 20%.

711 a) To decompress a duodenal stump after gastrectomy and gastro-jejunostomy.
b) To safeguard a difficult stump closure.
c) To enable post-operative alimentation.

N.B. Alexander-Williams recommends its use after any blind duodenal loop has been created in a gastric operation. The catheter balloon should be inflated with only 3 ml fluid. *(Proc. R.S.M. (1976)* *69* *847-848)*

712 a) Irritation/inflammation of the exit wound with or without frank infection.
b) Over-inflation of the balloon leading to partial obstruction of the duodenum (use only 3 ml of radio-opaque fluid).
c) Accidental deflation by medical or nursing staff.

N.B. Persistent fistula is rarely a problem.
(Alexander-Williams et al. Proc. R.S.M. (1976) *69* *847-848)*

713 Extra-dural: Lipoma, meningioma, neurofibroma, metastases.
Intra-dural: Extra-medullary - neurofibroma and meningioma.
Intra-medullary - glioma, ependymoma, vascular malformation.
N.B. Extra-dural metastatic tumours are by far the commonest.

714 Which is the best diagnostic way of visualising urethral valves?

715 Patients with malignant melanoma in the distal part of a limb who have histological evidence of lymph node spread, but no evidence of widespread or visceral metastases, often now receive isolated lumb perfusion. How much is the five year survival for this type of patient improved by this technique?

716 Stretching/laxity of the central slip of the extensor tendon of a finger leads to what deformity?

717 What are the dangers of passing a 'diagnostic catheter' in a case of possible rupture of the posterior urethra?

718 Define "keloid".

719 How common is a congenitally absent kidney?

720 What are the two main alternative operative procedures in the treatment of uncomplicated diverticular disease?

721 Classically 'cold' abscesses of the chest wall are secondary to what?

722 How would you treat such a case?

714 Voiding cystourethrograms.

715 Approximately 10% improvement only.

716 Boutonniere. (Flexed P.I.P. joint with hyperextended D.I.P. joint)

717 a) risk of making a partial tear worse, or completing it.
b) risk of introducing infection.
c) risk of misinterpreting the result: the fact that the catheter passes easily and 150 ml of clear, or slightly bloodstained, urine is evacuated does not exclude a full thickness tear of the urethra nor a ruptured bladder. If the catheter passes but no urine appears, the catheter may be in a normal but empty bladder, or it may lie in a ruptured bladder coiled up in the pelvis, or in the retropubic space.
d) If a catheter has already been passed, an aqueous cysto-urethrogram may be very helpful.

718 A scar within the skin that grows <u>beyond</u> the confines of the original wound. (Contrast the hypertrophic scar which is raised but which remains within the confines of the wound.)

719 1 in 1,400.

720 a) Colonic resection of the affected part.
b) Myotomy of the sigmoid or affected bowel.

721 Tuberculous intercostal lymphadenitis. The minority are due to Pott's of the spine or T.B. of the ribs or sternum.

722 Establish the diagnosis first if possible. Then start repeated aspirations through healthy skin with instillations of streptomycin. N.B. Start patient on triple chemotherapy. If this fails then display the extent of the abscess by lipiodol and X-ray, then perform surgery.

723 Who performed the second recorded bone transplant in history?

724 The workers in which industries are more prone to develop urothelial tumours?

725 What is the minimal number of Rads required to carry out an adequate mammogram?

726 What are the standard indications for performing primary flexor tendon suture in the injured hand when seen at night?

727 What is the differential diagnosis of a femoral hernia?

728 A cystic hygroma is a lymphangiomatous malformation which as its name implies often feels cystic. What physical sign must you demonstrate if possible?

729 In which sex, when and how does carcinoma of the tonsil present?

723 Cheiron who replaced Achilles' burned heel by the heel bone of a dead giant after Thetis dropped Achilles in a fire.
The first transplant is recorded in Genesis.

724 Chemical, rubber, cable industries if Beta naphthylamine is produced, and some plastics workers in the U.S.A.

725 The Manchester screening clinic quotes a minimal dose of 0.2 per breast. *(Leader B.M.J. (1977) 1 191-192.)*

726 This is a controversial subject ("No man's land" extends from the distal palmar crease to the D.I.P.J. crease).
a) The cut should not be in "no man's land".
b) A clean, unragged wound less than 6 hours old.
c) Minimal skin loss, and apparent ease of skin closure.
d) Absence of contraindications to postoperative immobilisation for up to 3 weeks.
e) An experienced hand surgeon available for back-up.

If the above do not apply, it is safer to explore the wound, tag the significant structures, close skin or obtain skin cover, and aim for delayed secondary tendon repair performed by an expert at leisure.

727 Inguinal hernia) It is remarkably easy to confuse
Saphena varix) these three unless you examine
Enlarged lymph node) the patient carefully.
Lipoma
Aneurysm
Psoas abscess or bursa
Ruptured adductor longus muscle

728 It transilluminates brilliantly.
(N.B. It may enlarge on coughing and may rarely be associated with macroglossia - always look inside the mouth.)

729 Mainly in elderly men (80%). They are often asymptomatic early on, then later when the faucial pillars are involved they have sore throat with pain, often severe, and referred to the ear associated with foul breath and bleeding. Dysphagia and trismus are late symptoms.

730 List some of the important principles in the reattachment of severed limbs or digits.

730 1. Dry-cool the severed part immediately, but do not place in direct contact with ice.
2. Prepare for immediate operation to reduce warm ischaemia time (which should be less than 6 hours).
3. Inform the blood transfusion service that you might need a lot of cross-matched blood, and send specimens immediately.
4. Irrigation with heparined saline of large arteries but not small ones. Avoid damaging vessels.
5. Avoid general anaesthesia is possible. A brachial block using marcaine can give satisfactory anaesthesia for up to eight hours. Have an anaesthetist available if your block fails.
6. Make sure that you have an assistant, and theatre staff prepared to work for up to twelve hours. (Re-establishing the circulation to the severed part may be only a minor part of the operation because all other structures should be repaired also to avoid secondary operations which could jeopardise the vascular anastomosis.)
7. At operation: Excise all devitalised tissue. Clean the stump without a tourniquet, identify and if necessary label all important structures with fine sutures. Clamp vessels at tip only.
8. Shorten and fix bones first to provide a stable limb for microvascular work.
9. Anastomose arteries first because this aids identification of veins in the severed part. Never suture vessels under tension. Tension can be avoided by either shortening bones or use of vein grafts, to bridge the gap.
10. If possible anastomose 2 to 3 veins for every artery repaired.
11. Anticoagulate only if the anastomoses are uncertain. Anticoagulation even for reattachment of a thumb can lead to enormous total blood loss. Low molecular weight dextrans and aspirin are preferable to heparinisation.
12. Perform elective fasciotomies where indicated to guard against effects of postoperative swelling.
13. Carry out primary nerve repairs under the operating microscope.
14. Repair tendons and muscle.
15. Adequate skin cover is vital, and skin flaps may be safer than skin grafts.

(B. McC. O'Brien, The Hand Vol. 6 No. 3 (1974) 217-228
" " " Annals of R.C.S. of E. (1976) 58 87-103)

731 What are the main types of skin flaps used in plastic surgery?

732 List the major complications of retropubic prostatectomy (excluding those associated with any major operation e.g. anaesthetic problems, D.V.T. etc.).

733 What is the usual earliest bladder disturbance in a patient with disseminated sclerosis?

734 Which organisms are commonly causes of infective cervical lymphadenitis in the U.K? How would you diagnose them?

735 What are the daily carbohydrate, fat, and protein requirements of the universal 70 kg man?

736 In whom is a thymectomy indicated?

737 If you are asked to comment on an X-ray of an apparently fractured patella what should you ask for before giving your opinion?

731 Random Pattern Flaps (random blood supply) - which may be divided into Transposition, Advancement, Rotation and Pedicled flaps.
Axial Pattern Flaps (blood supply runs along the axis of the flap, allowing a far greater length to breadth ratio than in random flaps.)
Free Flaps-usually an axial pattern flap transferred to its new site by microvascular surgery.

732 Operative Haemorrhage leading to technical difficulty.
Postoperative Haemorrhage (reactionary or secondary) which may lead to clot retention, catheter blockage, anaemia.
Infection +/- bacteraemia.
Epididymitis (some surgeons ligate the vasa prophylactically).
Suprapubic urinary fistula (rare).
Osteitis pubis (very rare).
Late postoperative Incomplete removal or regrowth.
Stricture (prostatic or bladder neck).
Incontinence.
Impotence.

733 Precipitency of micturition. The late sequelae of D.S. is usually retention with overflow which may be helped by detrusor stimulants. However, an in-dwelling catheter is usually required eventually.

734 Rubella: serology.
Haem. Strep. Group A: culture throat or primary lesion.
Toxoplasma: serology.
Mycobacteria (T.B. and atypical): Ziehl-Nielson stain and T.B. culture.

735 Approximately 300 g CHO, 60 g fat, 40 g protein.
(N.B. Multiply each by 4, 9, 4, respectively to give approximate calorie production.)

736 In myasthenics, particularly young females with a short history of myasthenia.
Patients with thymoma. (Pre-op. X.R.T. is often given.)
It has been advocated in renal transplant recipients.

737 An X-ray of the other side. The fracture may be a bi-partite patella which is, of course, usually symmetrical.

738 Outline the routine preparation of a patient for colonoscopy.

739 Medico-legal prudence and good clinical practice both suggest that you take which precautions before reducing a shoulder dislocation?

740 What are the common methods of treatment of achalasia of the oesophagus?

741 What chromosomal abnormality is often associated with a duodenal atresia?

742 In which cases of rectal cancer does downward extension of the tumour occur?

743 A man has a lesion on his forehead, which is 1 cm in diameter, has a raised rolled edge, ulcerated centre with crusting. What is the likely diagnosis and differential diagnosis?

744 What are the typical sites for intracranial meningiomata?

738 N.B. Never perform colonoscopy without barium enema first to identify potential hazards.
a) Empty the colon (low residue diet, cathartics, enemata).
b) Starve the patient for four hours prior to examination in case laparotomy is indicated if complications arise.
c) Have blood grouped for the patient in case transfusion is needed.
d) Give intravenous sedative and analgesic.
e) Perform colonoscopy with radiological screening available to locate colonoscope tip if necessary.

739 A neurological examination of the arm. Up to 70% of patients with a dislocated shoulder have a nerve lesion from the dislocation which, if undetected, before manipulation may afterwards be ascribed to your reduction. (Usually the circumflex nerve which, of course, supplies the deltoid shoulder joint and skin near it.

740 a) Self-bougienage (may be adequate in the mild case).
b) Forceful dilatation by pneumatic bag.
c) Cardiomyotomy (Heller's operation; probably the best treatment with reported 80% success rate. It carries the risk of reflux oesophagitis however.)
d) Anti-cholinergic drugs (not very effective in the long term).

741 Down's syndrome or Trisomy 21.

742 In cases where proximal lymphatics are obstructed. This is rare except in advanced cases. In most cases a 5 cm clearance below the macroscopic tumour will include all involved distal lymphatics. If the anal canal is involved extension downward occurs often. *(Morgan, Ann. R.C.S.Eng. (1965) 36 73-97)*

743 A nodular ulcerative basal cell carcinoma.
The differential diagnosis will include:- squamous cell carcinoma, malignant amelanotic melanoma, Bowen's intra-epithelial carcinoma.

744 Para-saggital, convexity, sphenoidal ridge, olfactory groove, suprasellar.

745 Differentiate irreducible, obstructed, incarcerated, strangulated hernia.

746 What are the classical signs of a malignant parotid tumour?

747 What are the main clinical features of the Plummer-Vinson syndrome?

748 How long can the average ileostomy patient keep his bag securely in place without having to change the whole appliance?

749 What symptoms are commonly regarded as being attributable to hiatus hernia?

750 What radiological improvement may be seen after successful MacMurray osteotomy for O.A. of the hip?

751 What kind of long term survival rates can be hoped for after successful resection in patients with carcinoma of the bronchus?

752 What is the name of the tube used for a calyco-pyelostomy?

745 Irreducible: Not reducible, bowel viable, hernia often contains only omentum.
Obstructed: Bowel is obstructed but viable, hernia may be irreducible but not necessarily.
Incarcerated: Strictly speaking this applies to the case where the lumen of that portion of colon occupying a hernial sac is blocked with faeces, in which event the scybalous contents should be indentable with a finger. The term is also used for an irreducible hernia containing viable bowel, but such usage is condemned by Bailey and Love.
Strangulated: Obstructed with impaired or absent blood supply to the contents.

746 A hard, irregular swelling with skin, VIIth nerve, and lymph node involvement. Facial nerve involvement in a parotid mass suggests malignancy.

747 A smooth tongue - not inflamed nor sore.
Spoon shaped finger nails which are often brittle.
Hypochromic anaemia.
Enlarged spleen) in some cases.
Achlorhydria)
Dysphagia usually due to spasm of upper oesophagus and post-cricoid web.

748 About 5-7 days. In some up to 10 days.

749 Heartburn, regurgitation, dysphagia, bleeding, vomiting, dyspepsia.

750 Widening of the narrow joint space (repair of the cartilage).
Clearance of subchondral bone sclerosis.
Disappearance of bone cysts.
N.B. Osteophytes seldom change.

751 At least one third are alive 5 years later and the occasional patient has survived over 30 years.
(Brock B.J.S. (1975) 62 1-5)

752 A Cummings tube.

753 What are the important complications of acute pancreatitis?

754 Most caecal diverticula are congenital in origin and can be distinguished histologically from diverticular disease. How?

755 What may be used in the (conservative) treatment of pneumatosis cystoides intestinales?

756 How valuable is the W.B.C. in the diagnosis of acute appendicitis?

757 What drug commonly used in ulcerative colitis has been recommended in Crohn's disease?

758 What is the commonest congenital anomaly of the upper renal tract?

759 List some of the presentations of polycystic kidneys in the adult?

753

Acute/Early	Chronic/Late
Dehydration	True abscess formation
Shock, possibly death	Pseudocyst
Septicaemia	Malabsorption
Acute renal failure	Drug addiction in relapsing pancreatitis
Gastric dilatation	
Reactivation of duodenal ulcer	
Hyperglycaemia associated with gross loss of islet tissue	
Basal collapse and pneumonia	

754 Congenital diverticula contain all layers of the intestinal wall. (They are usually solitary, occurring in younger patients than those with diverticulosis of the colon.) Acquired diverticula are herniations of mucosa between the muscle coats of the intestinal wall.

755 Oxygen therapy.

756 A very controversial topic. A leucocytosis of 12,000 or more with neutrophilia in excess of 75% supports the diagnosis. Levels lower than these merit review of the diagnosis but by no means exclude it. Suppurative appendicitis is regularly encountered with normal or low W.B.C.

757 Sulphasalazine (up to 3-4 gm daily). See *B.M.J. (1975)* 2 *297-298*. (Others include codeine phosphate, steroids and metronidazole.)

758 A duplicate renal pelvis. (It occurs in approximately 4% of the general population, *Bailey and Love*.)

759 Palpable loin mass.
Pain and tenderness in the renal angle (or elsewhere if the kidney is ectopic).
Haematuria.
Recurrent urinary tract infection.
Hypertension (found in 75% of patients over the age of 20 with polycystic kidneys).
Uraemia.

760 List some of the main features of rehabilitation of paraplegics.

761 How is carcinoma of the transverse colon treated?

762 Which nerve supplies the trapezius muscle?

763 How would you manage an undisplaced closed fracture of the patella with an intact quadriceps expansion? *(see leading article B.M.J. 23.8.75.)*

764 What are the main contraindications to upper gastro-intestinal endoscopy?

765 What are the features of the Peutz-Jegher's syndrome?

760 Aim is to return home to gainful employment.
Skin care: prevention of decubiti.
Mobilisation: prevention of contractures, wheelchair, transferring.
Activities of daily living: bladder and bowel care, dressing, driving, bathing.
Vocational training: assessment, training, placement.
Psychological counselling.
Treatment of complications: decubiti, urinary infections, spasticity.

761 Either: immediate resection with primary anastomosis
or excision of the tumour and mesentery with a spur colostomy
or caecostomy, proximal colostomy or ileostomy with later resection

762 11th - spinal accessory supplies motor branches and C3 and C4 proprioception.

763 After taking an adequate history, and carrying out a full examination, and performing the relevant investigations, including ...... (This is always a reasonable way to start a question about management tailoring the details to the particular topic.)
Treatment which is only one part of the question can be divided up into General, Local, Medical, Surgical, Urgent/Emergency and Elective, Complications and follow-up. Here under general, one could include treatment of other relevant disease or injuries, relief of pain, nursing care. Under local treatment: Aspiration of the knee joint, Robert Jones bandage or P.O.P. Cylinder. Early mobilisation and physiotherapy.
Surgery: patellectomy if pain persists due to uneveness of the healing fracture.

764 Poor condition of patient (especially cardio-respiratory disease); torrential bleeding.
Danger of cross-infection from the difficulty of sterilising the instrument especially in respect of hepatitis, T.B., and salmonellosis.

765 Speckled dark pigmentation of the lips associated with benign, single or multiple polyps usually in the jejunum, less commonly in the ileum, stomach, large bowel or even rectum. These may bleed and occasionally cause intussusception. Malignancy is very uncommon.

766 The aim of all treatment of congenital dislocation of the hip is to achieve and then maintain a congruous reduction thus allowing normal development of the femoral head and acetabulum. How is this done?

767 What electrolyte anomaly may occur in a patient suffering abdominal pain due to acute intermittent porphyria?

768 What are the commonly used instruments for exploring the C.B.D?

769 Which umbilical herniae in infants and children should be repaired?

770 Is there a non-familial form of (adenomatous) polyposis coli? (Polyposis coli = more than 100 polyps.)

771 Distinguish parathyroid adenoma from hyperplasia in terms of incidence, treatment, and further management of patients with primary hyperparathyroidism.

772 What should be checked (or done) immediately before repair of a large femoral hernia?

766 A. If the hip reduces easily and fully on gentle examination, splint in abduction with a frog P.O.P., followed by some more permanent form of splint e.g. Dennis Browne, von Rosen, until normal development occurs (usually 6-9 months).

B. If the hip will not reduce as in A, use gradual traction abducting legs for 2-3 weeks, then do A.

C. If B fails, open reduction, P.O.P., then splint.

D. If the hip is manifectly hopelessly unstable from the first, or if A, B, and C have all failed, proceed to innominate osteotomy.

767 A low serum sodium concentration due to inappropriate A.D.H. secretion.

768 Soft catheters and irrigation/Desjardins forceps bougies/ Bakes dilators/Scoops or fingers/Endoscopes.

769 a) Those which fail to decrease in size and close by school age. (Generally those whose defect is more than 1.5 cm diameter at the neck of the hernia.)
b) Rare cases causing pain or becoming incarcerated.

770 No. If there is no previous family history the patient has a new mutation and is likely to pass it on to his children. It has a dominant inheritance pattern with 80% penetrance and thus 40% of the children are likely to suffer from it, and 50% will pass on the gene. *(Bussey in Fam. Polyposis Coli, Baltimore 1975)*

771 Adenoma as a cause of primary hyperparathyroidism is much commoner than hyperplasia (about 80% : 20%). Adenoma should be removed in toto after checking all other parathyroids. Hyperplasia is treated by removal of as much tissue as is commensurate with the disease. The glands which remain should be marked with clips in case more tissue needs to be excised later. Patients with primary hyperplasia may be suffering from the multiple endocrine adenomatosis syndrome type I and this should be sought.

772 Make sure the bladder is empty, if necessary catheterise. N.B. This is sometimes advisable with a very large direct inguinal hernia.

773 List some of the features to be sought or considered in the history and examination of a possible 'battered' baby.

774 How are B.C.G. injections in 'immunotherapy' thought to work?

775 Vagotomy and pyloroplasty is probably not a good operation for gastric bleeding due to erosive gastritis. Why?

776 What are the important features of mastitis carcinomatosa?

773 In the History: Inconsistency or implausibility in the explanation of the cause of the 'accident', with associated frequently poor history of previous accidents. The parent(s) may be evasive or unco-operative. Parents may show an abnormal attitude to the injury. Delay between injury and presentation at hospital or G.P. surgery is very suspicious.

On immediate examination: There may be evidence of unexplained fractures, bruises, lacerations, burns etc. The child may be mal-nourished, dirty, with napkin-area dermatitis. Child's behaviour may be very withdrawn. Bruises on the shins are common in children but on the backs of the legs are often due to 'battering'.

Special points to look for: Torn frenum of upper lip, mucosal petechiae ....

Observation over several days: Child may start to thrive in hospital, but behaviour may be noticeably altered by parental visits.

X-ray examination: Old healed, or new fractures; periosteal thickening of long bones; separation or widening of cranial sutures; metaphyseal or diaphyseal new bone formation; separation of epiphyses.

774 The B.C.G. is thought to act both as a non-specific activator of macrophages thus aiding their 'agressiveness' towards tumour cells, and also as a stimulant of tumour-specific immunity. *(Bart et al. Annals N.Y. Acad. Sci. (1976) 277, 60-93.*

775 The mortality is high. (One figure quoted is 25-33%). Continued bleeding is common. Bile reflux which may exacerbate the condition is facilitated. A Billroth I may be a better procedure. *(Reynolds, Annals R.C.S. Eng. (1974) 55 213-225.)*

776 It is rare. (2% of breast carcinoma) Commonly mostly in pregnancy or lactation. Breast painful. Nipple often retracted. Skin red, oedematous, and warm. (Dermal lymphatics involved.) Axillary glands usually negative. May be mistaken for abscess, but does not show pyrexia nor leucocytosis. Early mastectomy is desirable. Most have very poor prognosis.

777 Percutaneous electrical cordotomy is believed to be an effective method of relieving intractable pain. It is commonly performed at either the C1-C2 level, the latter avoiding the problem of apnoea occurring in sleep. Which tracts are destroyed by the method and what are the side effects?

778 Describe in outline the Oschner-Sherren regime of management of appendicitis. It is much used nowadays?

779 What is the risk of a premenopausal patient with a breast carcinoma developing a second primary in the other breast?

780 What nerve lesions cause a full claw hand?

781 Is carcinoma of the pancreas commoner in diabetics?

782 In which patients and in which situations is it difficult to decide whether to perform anterior resection or an abdomino-perineal resection of a tumour and what may be an acceptable alternative procedure?

783 Is it justified to remove a normal looking Meckel's diverticulum, incidental to another intra-abdominal procedure?

777 The antero-lateral tracts at the upper end of the spinal cord thus producing analgesia on the opposite site of the body. There is also loss of heat and cold sensation. Care must be taken to avoid motor or bladder function loss. Late dysaesthesia may occur. Pain is usually controlled for some months and the procedure is best confined to the terminally ill.

778 The patient is nursed sitting upright to achieve drainage of exudate into the pelvis; intensive antibiotic therapy; nil by mouth except sips of water increased if patient's condition improves after 24 hours. Continuous monitoring of pulse and temperature, avoidance of strong analgesics, examination of patient gently by one person, the surgeon. If temperature, pulse, or pain increases at any time then operation *(Hamilton Bailey)*.
It is rarely used because the complication rate (including mortality) is so high. It may have to be used occasionally in special circumstances (e.g. on board ship).

779 There is an increased risk of 5 times the rate for controls, overall. *(Davis-Christopher Textbook of Surgery 11th Ed. 1977 Saunders p. 657.)*

780 Loss of C8 and T1 fibres to the hand e.g. combined median and ulnar division, Klumpkes paralysis, medial cord injuries.

781 Yes. Ten times commoner than in the general population, although diabetes only occasionally develops in a patient with carcinoma of the pancreas. *(Bailey and Love.)*

782 Cases of well differentiated middle third tumours of the rectum - i.e. 7.5 - 12 cm from the anal verge. Anterior resection may be technically very difficult if the lower limit of resection lies at or only just above the pelvic floor. It is also more difficult in the male and the obese. An alternative operation is the anal pull-through. *(B.J.S. (1965) 52 323.)*

783 No. See reference: *Soltero and Bill 1976 Am. J. Surg. 132 168.*
The Majority of Meckel's diverticula that bleed do so in the first three years of life.

784 Describe the standard above-knee myoplastic amputation. (Operative technique.)

785 At what time is a woman at greatest risk of developing pelvic sepsis from an intra-uterine contraceptive device?

786 What are the main contraindications to circumcision in the infant or child?

787 When did Fallot first describe his tetralogy?

788 Name some causes of free blood in the peritoneal cavity?

789 In acute pancreatitis when does the calcium level generally fall?

784 Pre-op. explanation to patient of immediate post-op. positioning, movements and mobilisation. Mark the side. Pre-op. penicillin. G.A. Supine position on operating table. Check the side, prep. and drape. Mark out flaps with Bonney's Blue. Equal anterior and posterior flaps. Skin flaps are turned back to 8 inches above the knee joint. Identify, ligate and divide the long saphenous vein as a separate step. Marker sutures are placed in each main muscle group about 6 inches above the level of the knee joint. Divide the muscles down to bone just above the patella, lift them up from the bone by sharp dissection to approximately 7 inches above the knee joint. Ligate vessels. Pull down nerves and divide, secure any bleeding vessels (there is often a large one with the sciatic nerve) and allow them to retract. Form a periosteal flap (3 inches below the level of the intended bone section) from the anterior bone surface. Saw through the femur 10 inches below greater trochanter (approximately 7 inches above the level of the knee joint). Lay the periosteum over the bone end, then pull muscles down so that the marker sutures are in line with the bone end. Trim the muscles and suture opposing groups to each other i.e. adductors to abductors and then quadriceps to hamstrings. Trim the skin flaps, and suture without tension with suction drains. Apply firm wool or soft padding with crepe bandage. Some surgeons enclose the end in plaster of Paris. Discuss post-op. management and rehabilitation, complications early and late.

785 During the first 2-3 weeks following insertion of the I.U.C.D. However, she still has a five-fold higher risk of pelvic sepsis than a woman without an I.U.C.D.

786 The presence of hypospadias.
The child being unfit for anaesthesia.
N.B. Most are unnecessary.

787 1888.
Pulmonary stenosis, R.V.H., V.S.D., over-riding of aorta.

788 Ruptured: ectopic pregnancy, luteal cyst, abdominal viscus (spleen, liver, bowel or their mesenteries) retroperitoneal structure with breech in peritoneum i.e. kidney/aneurysm.

789 About the 5th to 8th day.

790 Which childhood fractures may need internal fixation?

791 In the treatment of hypoparathyroidism and in particular the hypocalcaemia after thyroid or parathyroid operations which drugs may be used?

792 In the lung, which"ectopic" hormones is a squamous cell carcinoma likely to produce in contrast to an oat cell carcinoma?

793 Most patients with a short gut syndrome can be managed medically. What will this treatment be? What may the surgical treatment be in cases of failure of medical treatment?

794 What is the approximate mortality of acute pancreatitis in England? (N.B. It varies according to cause. In some countries i.e. U.S.A. and South Africa, alcoholism is a very common cause.)

795 Of those with carcinoid tumour(s), which patients develop the syndrome of flushing, intestinal disturbance, and right-sided heart disease?

790 Very few childhood fractures require open reduction and internal fixation because:-
(i) children's bones remodel, and less perfect reductions are acceptable.
(ii) children tolerate traction and P.O.P. well.
(iii) one tries to avoid internal fixation on growing bones.

If maintenance of a satisfactory reduction is impossible by closed means, internal fixation must be used. The commonest sites are around the elbow viz. supracondylar humoral, radial neck and medial epicondylar fractures.

791 As an emergency; slow intravenous calcium gluconate.
In urgent cases: calcium sandoz tabs. 1-2 q.d.s. + A.T.10 (which is 25 Dihydrotachysterol) 3 ml daily until calcium appears in the urine.
Long term: Vitamin D with a loading dose of 400,000 units, maintenance 150,000 units/day.

792 Squamous cell carcinoma: parathyroid like hormone.
Oat cell carcinoma: A.C.T.H., M.S.H., A.D.H. like hormones.
(Adenocarcinoma: gonadotropin)
Omenn and Wilkins 1970, J. Thor. & Cardio Vascular Surgery, 59 877.

793 Low fat non-residue diet and added medium chain triglycerides. Cholestyramine may be used to leach out the bile acids, which can be responsible for "Choleretic diarrhoea". (Excess bile acids entering the colon). Drugs such as Codeine or Lomotil may slow down transit time.
Reversal of a very critical length of small bowel (usually 7-14 cm). The distal end of the residual small bowel is used to fashion the reversed loop.
(Leader B.M.J. (1975) 2 709-710)

794 Over a twenty year period at Bristol it was 17%.
(Trapnell and Duncan B.M.J. (1975) 2 179-183.)

795 Those with hepatic or general metastases. When the tumour is small and the liver intact the vasoactive hormones are cleared from the circulation too rapidly to cause symptoms.

796 What are the most useful investigations in the diagnosis of a renal mass in the newborn?

797 What are the main available methods of humidification of air for a tracheostomy patient in the post-operative period?

798 Which types of intestinal polyps are believed to be pre-cancerous?

799 Name some causes of cirrhosis in children and infants.

800 Should one perform oesophagoscopy on a child suspected of swallowing corrosive?

801 What is the canal of Nuck?

802 What is glove powder made of nowadays?

796 Initially a radioisotope scan. If an I.V.U. is performed on a baby less than a few days old, the excretion is usually poor and inadequate information is gained for a higher radiation dose. If a scan is used together with an ultrasound examination, the cause of the renal mass can usually be ascertained; e.g. multicystic kidney, hydronephrosis.

797 a) Nursing the patient in a humidified atmosphere.
b) Heat and moisture exchangers applied directly to the tracheostomy tube.
c) Bubble humidifiers heated and thermostatically controlled.
d) Mechanical or ultrasonic nebulisers of heated water.

798 Definitely pre-malignant: villous adenoma, familial polyposis coli.
Probably pre-malignant: papillary adenoma, esp. if wider than 1 cm diameter.
Not pre-malignant: metaplastic polyps, juvenile polyps, Peutz-Jeghers polyps.

799 Congenital hepatic fibrosis and erythro blastosis foetalis.
Infective: viral hepatitis.
Cardiac cirrhosis.
Nutritional: in vegetarians, protein deficiency +/- Kwashiokor Galactosaemia.
Atresia of the bile ducts: occurs in only those surviving a few months.

800 Yes, as soon as possible after the accident, to assess degree and extent of damage. The risk of perforation by such instrumentation is least in the first twenty-four hours. Oedema should be distinguished from slough which is usually white. The former is seldom associated with later strictures the latter frequently. Oesophagoscopy may have to be repeated a few weeks after the accident. Several authorities recommend the early use of steroids. *(Haller J. A., et al (1971) J. Ped. Surg. 6 579.)*

801 The persistent processus vaginalis in the female which lies in the inguinal canal and accompanies the round ligament of the uterus.

802 Maize starch.

803 How would you advise a patient who was found to have gall stones on a plain abdominal X-ray who had never suffered symptoms referable to the gall bladder?

804 Why is the diagnosis of actinomycosis of the ileo-caecal region often missed?

805 Why is a saphenous vein by-pass considered to be better than popliteal endarterectomy in the treatment of femoro-popliteal disease?

806 The superficial inguinal pouch lies between which two anatomical layers?

807 What is white bile?

808 What distinguishes histologically a lentigo malignum from malignant melanoma?

803 This is a controversial topic. Statistically, 50% will develop symptoms, and about one third will need a cholecystectomy. Selection of which individual is likely to benefit is difficult, but a non-functioning gall bladder on cholecystogram makes it more likely, and thus a cholecystogram may be worthwhile if asymptomatic cholelithiasis is discovered by chance. The chances of a person dying from carcinoma of the gall bladder (associated with cholelithiasis) are less than from routine surgery. Most surgeons recommend cholecystectomy for fit patients under 55 years.
(B.M.J. (1975) Leader 1, 415, letter Russell and Dudley 2, 277).

804 It is often forgotten, as a possible cause of an appendix mass. The organism is best grown anaerobically and unless anaerobic culture is requested and commenced immediately at the time of operation it may never be grown. Actinomycosis is sensitive to penicillin and other antibiotics which may be given to a patient with a wound infection and thus the 'sulphur granules' may never appear in the pus which merely contains a lot of chronic inflammatory cells.

805 a) The distal popliteal artery is usually too small or narrow to do a satisfactory endarterectomy. (The risk of raising an intimal flap at the distal end is considerable and closure without narrowing almost impossible.)
b) The disease is seldom localised to a short segment.
c) The five year survival figures for by-pass procedure are better.

806 Scarpa's Fascia (membranous layer of the superficial fascia) and the external oblique aponeurosis.

807 Mucus only, virtually no bile salts; it occurs immediately after the release of relatively long standing biliary obstruction, and in mucoceles.

808 Although there is much junctional activity with a disorganised epidermis there is no dermal invasion in a lentigo malignum. It is thus an 'in-situ' form of malignant melanoma. It can progress and about one third become frankly malignant but this is a late phenomenon.

809 Give a list of the important points in the pathology of medulloblastoma.

810 The paper on suturing by Jenkins *(B.J.S. 1976 63, 873)* strongly suggests that the likely cause of most cases of burst abdominal wound is what?

811 Give a list of the causes of hyperthyroidism.

812 In health, what is the concentration of O_2 and CO_2 in expired air?

813 What tumours are associated with amyloid disease?

809 Incidence : About 5% of all gliomata. One of the commoner cerebral tumours of childhood.
Aetiology : Unknown.
Sex : Twice as common in males.
Geography : No geographical predominance or racial association.
Age : 50% occur under the age of 10 years.
Macroscopic: Soft greyish pink in colour.
Microscopic: Sheets of round cells, scanty cytoplasm, loose connective tissue stroma.
Site : Subtentorial. Commonest in midline cerebellum and 4th ventricle.
Spread : Along C.S.F. pathways, seldom outside C.N.S.
Prognosis : Usually poor. With radiotherapy about 30% survive at 10 years.
(Bloom H.J.B. et al. Am J. Roentg 105: 43, 1969.)

810 The method of suturing the wound:
Distension of the abdomen may increase the length of the wound by 30%. Interrupted suturing may lead to potential gaps between sutures and increased tension on those sutures. With continuous suturing the tension on the suture line rises exponentially with rise in intra-abdominal pressure. Jenkins recommends that a continuous suture should be 4 x length of the wound. Bites should be deep and less than 1 cm apart.

811 a) Diffuse toxic goitre (as in Grave's disease).
b) Toxic nodular goitre: multinodular, toxic adenoma, or nodular goitre with Grave's disease.
c) Excess T.S.H.: Pituitary tumour
Choriocarcinoma/hydatidiform mole
Embryonal testicular carcinoma
d) Extraneous thyroid hormone:

Exogenous	Endogenous
Intentionally factitious	Metastatic thyroid carcinoma
Overenthusiastic therapy	Struma ovarii
During T_3 suppression test	

Jod-Baselow disease (thyroid hormone induced).
e) Thyroiditis associated: subacute, Hashimoto's, irradiation, T.S.H. administration.

812 O_2 16%, CO_2 4%.

813 Chronic inflammation (including T.B.), myeloma, Hodgkins, renal cell carcinoma.

814 What are the causes of extra-hepatic portal vein obstruction?

815 Apart from the relatively common and usually transient post-operative or post-partum causes, acute retention of urine in women may be due to which other causes or diseases?

816 What are the basic clinical signs of an A.S.D. (Atrial septal defect)?

817 List some of the commoner causes of post-operative jaundice.

818 What is the meaning of a T_1 tumour of the breast?

814 Sepsis leading to thrombosis:- via umbilicus in neonate;
after pyelo-phlebitis;
in association with multiple liver abscesses.

Thrombosis:- after an exchange transfusion in the neonate;
in association with 'thrombophlebitis migrans;'
due to polycythaemia or leukaemia.

Directly:- tumour of liver, Porta Hepatis, pancreas, stomach, kidney or colon by compression or invasion.

815 Gynaecological
Pelvic mass
Prolapse
Pessary
Vulval haematoma

Neurological
D.S.
Traumatic paraplegia
Sacral agenesis
Cerebral metastasis
'Hysteria'

Rectal
Faecal impaction
Severe colitis

Urological
Urethral stenosis
Urethral inflammation
Bladder neck obstruction

816 Slight right ventricular enlargement.
Marked pulsation of the pulmonary artery in 2nd and 3rd intercostal space.
Pulmonary systolic murmur (a 'flow' murmur).
Fixed split second sound in pulmonary area (unaffected by respiration).

817 Hepatic/biliary surgery: retained stones, oedema/spasm of the ampulla, operative damage to common bile duct.
Anaesthesia: Halothane (hepatocellular damage).
Blood transfusion: Bilirubin overload from stored blood in the presence of depressed liver function, mismatched transfusion.
Infection: haemolysis ++.
Unexplained cholestatic jaundice. Drugs etc.
Exacerbation of pre-existing liver disease - e.g. cirrhosis

818 A tumour of 2 cm or less in its greatest dimension.
Divisible into
T_{1a} = Tumour without deep fixation.
T_{1b} = Tumour with fixation to deep fascia or pectoral muscle.
(Clinical Oncology by Horton & Hill, 1977 Saunders p.46)

819 What are the typical signs and symptoms of a gastric volvulus? What is the treatment?

820 What factors have been shown statistically to affect the mortality of chronic peptic ulcer haemorrhage?

821 Which muscles does C.5 spinal segment subserve?

822 What vital structures must be safe-guarded when excising a cervical rib using a superior approach?

819 The patient may give history of recurrent attacks of upper abdominal pain with distension accompanied by retching. Occasionally the volvulus fails to reduce itself causing sudden pain often severe beginning generally after a meal and gradually worsening. Shock may ensue. Patient may retch producing small amounts of bileless frothy vomit. There is frequently a resonant swelling in the upper abdomen and a nasogastric tube often cannot be passed. On X-ray there is an enormous gastric air shadow.
Early exploration is indicated, deflate the stomach using the puncture site for gastrostomy, untwist the stomach, and perform a gastropexy to the anterior abdominal wall, after separating the greater curve from the omentum and colon.

820 Many studies have highlighted several factors in the history, signs on examination and treatment that affected the outcome.
1. Age of patient: mortality rises rapidly after the age 45 years.
2. Number of bleeding episodes: mortality doubles if haemorrhage stops and then starts again as a new episode, and continuous uncontrolled bleeding carries a worse prognosis still.
3. B.P. on presentation: the lower the B.P. the higher the mortality.
4. Number of units of blood transfused: the more the worse.
5. Pulse on presentation: mortality rises with increasing pulse rate from 80/min to 100/min.
6. Type of surgery: Polya gastrectomy although having a better long-term cure rate carried a higher operative mortality than vagotomy and pyloroplasty.
7. Presence of co-existent disease i.e. cardio-respiratory.

821 Biceps, Brachialis, Brachioradialis, Coracobrachialis, Deltoid, part of supinator, Pectoralis Major, Rhomboids, Serratus Anterior, Spinati, Subscapularis, Teres Minor.

822 Phrenic nerve.
Subclavian artery and vein.
Brachial plexus especially the supra-scapular nerve.
Cervical sympathetic trunk.
Pleura.

823 What is usually regarded as the best palliative procedure for gastric carcinoma? (N.B. many surgeons feel that all operations for stomach cancer are palliative as the 5 year survival is very low. Sarcomata, lymphomata and the rare metastatic carcinomata have a slightly better prognosis.)

824 What are the pathological features of a bladder infected with S.Haematobium?

825 How soon would you expect a confident bacteriological report that an empyema which you have just tapped is sterile?

826 The introduction of the ventriculo-atrial shunt for hydrocephalus stimulated a policy of 'treatment for all' in the management of spina bifida, in some units. What was the outcome of this policy?

827 Name some common drugs which alter the action of Warfarin.

823 Resection of the tumour beyond the macroscopic line of spread so that the patient dies from hepatic metastases rather than gastric obstruction etc. If resection is impossible then exclusion gastro-jejunostomy may have to be employed.

824 a) In schistosomiasis the accumulation of eggs submucosally may appear as pseudotubercles, or pearls (similar to true tuberculous tubercles).
b) Ulceration and papillomatous lesions may develop on the mucosa leading to secondary infection and acute cystitis.
c) Fibrotic scarring of mucosa and underlying wall, with 'sandy patches' (calcification of the shells of the ova leading to an outline of the bladder on plain radiograph).
d) The intramural ureter may stenose causing hydronephrosis or reflux.
e) Late complications include squamous carcinoma especially at the trigone, and its onset is particularly difficult to identify as many of the patients already have intermittent haematuria.

825 Only after at least 5 days. Many anaerobes are slow growing, and a microbiologist will require this length of time to exclude their presence unless he has access to gas-liquid chromatography when absence of branched or longchained fatty acids will permit their earlier exclusion. *(Noone and Rogers, J. Clin. Microbiol. (1976) 29 652-656.)*

826 In a phrase - great controversy. Lorber in 1971 showed that treating all spina bifida cases resulted in a high mortality in those surviving at birth, and high morbidity of those not dying soon after birth, i.e. prolonged handicap from gross paralyses, deformity of the legs, kyphosis, scoliosis, urinary incontinence with hydronephrosis, chronic pyelonephritis and hypertension. Most centres now follow policies of selection.
(Lorber, Devl. Med. Child Neurol. (1971) 13 279-303.)

827 Barbiturates, Antacids, Corticosteroids, oral contraceptives, Vitamin K, Phenylbutazone, Indomethazine, Ibrufen, Penicillin, Ampicillin, Tetracycline, Alcohol, liquid paraffin.

828 In an emergency, what types of blood are available, and how long can you expect it to take for these to be issued?

829 How should you describe a 'lump'?

830 Which antibiotics should have their dosage modified in acute renal failure (if dialysis has not been commenced)?

831 Instrumentation of the oesophagus is one of the commoner causes of rupture, less common now with the use of fibre-optic flexible instruments. Prognosis is related to early recognition and treatment. Cervical rupture is associated with pyrexia, supra-clavicular tenderness, spasm of the sterno-mastoid, and surgical emphysema. A thoracic rupture causes deep mediastinal pain, and rupture at the cardia causes epigastric pain. What immediate investigations should be carried out on a suspected rupture?

828 In a catastrophic crisis, 0 neg. blood (screened for irregular antibodies) is available immediately and can be given safely to all patients.

If the patient's blood group is known, blood of the same ABO group and rhesus type can be given without cross-match but the procedure carries a significant risk.

In an urgent situation, allow ten minutes for the specimen to clot and the serum to be separated. ABO emergency grouping with partial rhesus typing takes a further five minutes. Thus fifteen minutes are needed for grouping and typing.

An emergency cross-match takes 30 minutes after the preceding grouping. Thus 45 minutes should be allowed for this.

A full cross-match takes 2½ hours.

829 By its:- Site, shape, size, surface, sound (bruit).
Consistency - solid/cystic and if emptyable.
Colour - blood/pigment.
Temperature and transilluminability.
Attachments - superficial/deep and diff. mobility.
Associated lymph nodes or lesions.
Any distant effects.

830 a) All aminoglycosides. Gentamicin, tobromycin, streptomycin, kanamycin, neomycin. (Ototoxicity and nephrotoxicity)
b) High dosage penicillins. (Neurotoxicity.)
c) All tetracyclines (except doxycycline). (Make renal failure worse.)
d) All cephalosporins. (Nephro and neurotoxicity.)
e) Chloramphenical. (Accumulation of toxic metabolites.)
f) Trimethoprim. (Antifolate activity.)

831 Full blood count, blood culture, X-ray of neck, chest or abdomen as appropriate, and dilute barium swallow*.
Tanner recommends conservative treatment with antibiotics only for cervical rupture and antibiotics and early repair for all the others.
(* Barium should be used in preference to gastrograffin in the chest.)

832 Which lung function tests are commonly done as a pre-operative assessment prior to thoracic surgery?

833 What are the chief indications for drainage of the peritoneal cavity?

834 What factors appear to predispose to or are certainly associated with a burst abdominal wound?

835 What solutions may be used to wash out the bowel pre-operatively just prior to anastomosis in an attempt to prevent implantation of tumour cells at the site of anastomosis?

836 In which age group of women is medullary carcinoma of the breast typically found?

832 a) V.C.
b) $F.E.V_1$.
c) P.E.F.R. (Peak expiratory flow rate) with Wright flow meter.
d) Assess the effect of a bronchodilator on these after ten minutes (i.e. 0.16 mg Isoprenaline) if either a,b,c are availabe.
e) Blood gases.
f) The effect of exercise on these measurements is helpful, if any of the others are abnormal.

833 Controversial, but most surgeons would agree with the following:-
1. The presence of an abscess or free purulent fluid.
2. When haemostasis is in doubt.
3. When bile leakage is anticipated.
4. When the integrity of the bowel is in doubt or has been interrupted, e.g. an anastomosis, or oversewing.
If in doubt: drain, except possibly in the presence of inoperable carcinoma with malignant ascites where drainage may allow implantation of carcinoma in the drainage wound and later fungation and breakdown of the abdominal wall.

834 Upper abdominal incisions.
Suture of wounds under tension. (Mass-Suture technique reduces incidence.)
Low Hb. level. (under 11 gms%)
Hypoproteinaemia. (under 6.5 gms%)
Pre-operative ileus or peritonitis or debilitation (especially disseminated carcinoma).
Obesity.
Coughing, vomiting, post-op. ileus.
Wound infection.

835 1:500 mercuric chloride
distilled water
thiotepa
noxythiolin
cetrimide
(Naunton-Morgan Proc. R.S.M. (1957) 50)

836 Those aged 25-35 years and usually under 50 years. Medullary carcinomata represent approximately 7% of all breast carcinomata, and carry a better long term prognosis than other types.
(Bloom et Al B.M.J. (1970) 3 181-187)

837 Give an outline summary of the management of a major upper gastro-intestinal bleed.
(N.B. the answer we have given is very brief and serves only as an example of the barest outline. The question is asked mainly to encourage you to sort out the answer in your own mind so that when you actually reach the green-baize table you will be able to rattle it all off with panache.)

838 Is X.R.T. indicated for carcinoma of the oesophagus?

839 What effect on the five year survival does the presence of involved lymph nodes make at the initial presentation of malignant melanoma?

837 Resuscitate first. (Fluid immediately i.e. plasma/dextran and then blood replacement.) Remember to cross-match sufficient blood to allow for a subsequent bleed.
History and examination: with reference especially to past G.I. tract symptoms, operations, drug ingestion - steroid/anti inflammatory etc.
Gauge speed and quantity of blood replacement by C.V.P./ urine output/Hb., P.C.V. etc. Assess need for digitalisation and diuretics.
Correct as far as possible electrolyte disturbance.
Attempt early definitive diagnosis by endoscopy/radiology.
If lesion is mucosal (oesophagitis/Mallory W./acute erosions) aim to treat conservatively because most stop spontaneously.
Peptic ulcer: Avoid delay, especially in the old, and those with big bleeds, and also those patients with no previous history who are too often treated conservatively for too long.
Duodenal ulcer: Underrun the ulcer and do the ulcer operation you know best (Truncal/Selective Vagotomy + Pyloroplasty).
Gastric ulcer/Erosive Gastritis: unresponsive to medical therapy Billroth I partial gastrectomy. Neoplasm - attempt definitive operation where practicable.
Bleeding varices: Initial conservatism with blood replacement/Vit. K, vasopressin/Senstaken-B Tube. If these fail either sclerosants or surgery. (Know the alternatives.

838 Yes, in some cases. Lower one third tumours are often columnar cell in type and radio-resistant. Upper and middle one third may benefit if inoperable. Surgery or other palliative procedures are indicated otherwise.
(Cancer - Del Regato. Chap. 13, p. 455-458 (1977) St. Louis, Mosby.)

839 Nodes clinically and microscopically: 5 yr.survival

clinically	microscopically	5 yr. survival
negative	negative	56%
negative	positive	30%
positive	negative	27%
positive	positive	10%

(Gumpert and Harris Ann. Surg. (1974) 179 105-108) (306 patients 90% follow up)

840 Which two organisms are commonly responsible for post-operative pneumonia? Select three antibiotics for their treatment.

841 Work out the topics you would discuss in an essay on the use (and abuse) of surgical drainage.

842 What are the fluid requirements per kg/24 hrs. without excess fluid loss of a baby:?
(i) 2 days old
(ii) 1 week old
(iii) 8 weeks old

840 (Staph. aureus is a rare cause of such problems unless aspiration has occurred; anaerobes are unlikely.)
The commonest organisms are:

	Pneumococcus (Str.pneumoniae)	Haemophilus influenzae
Benzyl penicillin	OK	2 Megaunits qds
Ampicillin, amoxycillin	OK	OK
Co-trimoxazole	probably OK	Resistant
Oxytetracycline	0-5% resist.	5-10% resist.
Gentamicin, tobramycin	inactive	poor sputum penetr. not used alone
Erythromycin	OK	usually inadequate alone
Lincomycin, clindomycin	OK	inactive
Metronidazole	inactive	inactive

(Philip and Spencer 1974 B.M.J. I 359-361)

841 There are many ways of approaching this topic, but it is probably helpful to split the answer into as many headings as possible so that you will not forget too much.
For example:-
Distinguish internal from external drainage.
" cavity from pure wound drainage.
Discuss indications and then contraindications in clean and septic cases, giving examples.
Types of drain used:- Static, suction, under-water, tube or solid.
Materials:- rubber, plastic, gauze.
Size and siting of drains.
Fixation,
Duration of drainage. 'Shortening'.
Complications:- foreign body reaction, introduction of infection, perforation of viscus or artery
Give special examples:-
Cerebral abscess
Hydrocephalus
Pneumothorax, empyema
Biliary T-Tubc
Pyelostomy
Urinary

842 (i) 85ml/kg/24 hr.
(ii)150ml/kg/24 hr.
(iii)100ml/kg/24 hr.

843 Briefly outline the management of a severely burned patient from the time of arrival in Casualty.

843 In the Casualty Department
Establish time, cause of burn. Estimate areas of full, partial thickness, superficial burn if possible. Search for signs of inhalation of smoke. Establish baselines Hb., P.C.V., Electrolytes. X-match blood. Consult burns expert. Start prophylactic penicillin. I.V. fluid replacement: if possible use a patent vein in area of full thickness burn (painless). Cover burned areas loosely with sterile towels and transfer patient to Burns Unit. N.B. burns of over 10% in children up to 15 years old, 15% in adults require fluid replacement.

In Burns Unit
Check history and repeat examination; draw and photograph burn.
Dressing Open technique ± topical antiseptic agents
Closed technique: Paraffin gauze/Pig skin/ Artificial skin.
Analgesia requirements minimal once wound is dressed.
Fluid replacement Assess initially by formula (Brookearmy/ Evans/Odstock/Muir & Barclay) then by frequent clinical assessment + Pulse, B.P., Resp., Blood Gases, P.C.V., Urine Output and osmolality, Hb'uria, Proteinuria, etc. (Shock phase lasts for about 48 hours.)
Control of Infection Sterile wound dressing technique. Wound swabs. Avoid prophylactic antibiotics except penicillin. Blood culture if indicated.
Surgery Conservative: Await separation of slough (about three weeks) - split skin grafts to healthy granulations. Aggressive: Early 'tangential' excision (about 3-7 days)- meshed or ordinary skin grafts.
Physiotherapy Keep all joints mobile to reduce stiffness and oedema. Use plastic bag to cover hand and feet burns. Chest physiotherapy. Splints (Dynamic or fixed) where indicated.
Rehabilitation and Follow-up Skin care. Hypertrophic scars: steroids/pressure garments. Surgery: release of contractures with skin grafts or skin flaps, Z-plasties etc. N.B. Frequent talks to patient and relatives from the outset are essential part of management.
Complications Chest infection, D.V.T., Septicaemia, Renal Failure, Curling's Ulcer.

*(I. F. K. Muir & T. L. Barclay, Burns and Their Treatment, 2nd Ed. (1974) Lloyd-Luke.
Evans, E.I., Annals of Surgery, 122 693 (1954)
Laing, J.E. & Harvey, J, The Management and Nursing of Burns. Unibook, English University Press.)*

INDEX OF QUESTIONS

INDEX OF QUESTIONS

INDEX OF QUESTIONS

INDEX OF QUESTIONS

INDEX OF QUESTIONS

INDEX OF QUESTIONS

INDEX OF QUESTIONS

INDEX OF QUESTIONS

INDEX OF QUESTIONS

INDEX OF QUESTIONS

INDEX OF QUESTIONS

INDEX OF QUESTIONS

INDEX OF QUESTIONS

INDEX OF QUESTIONS

INDEX OF QUESTIONS